# GENDER, HEALTH AND HEALTHCARE

*For our girls, Halina and Lily Pie*

*Also for Gabrielle White who helped make possible the start of my feminist journey and for Dr Joyce Cavaye, my intellectual collaborator and friend*

# Gender, Health and Healthcare

## Women's and Men's Experience of Health and Working in Healthcare Roles

JACQUELINE H. WATTS
*The Open University, UK*

ASHGATE

Published by
Ashgate Publishing Limited
Wey Court East
Union Road
Farnham
Surrey, GU9 7PT
England

Ashgate Publishing Company
110 Cherry Street
Suite 3-1
Burlington, VT 05401-3818
USA

www.ashgate.com

**British Library Cataloguing in Publication Data**
A catalogue record for this book is available from the British Library

**The Library of Congress has cataloged the printed edition as follows:**
Watts, Jacqueline H., author.
Gender, health and healthcare : women's and men's experience of health and working in healthcare roles / by Jacqueline H. Watts.
p. cm.
Includes bibliographical references and index.
ISBN 978-1-4094-6836-3 (hardback) – ISBN 978-1-4094-6837-0 (ebook) – ISBN 978-1-4094-6838-7 (epub)
I. Title. [DNLM: 1. Gender Identity. 2. Health Personnel. 3. Health Behavior. 4. Health Promotion. 5. Health Status. 6. Sexism. W 21]
RA776.5
613–dc23

2014041048

ISBN 9781409468363 (hbk)
ISBN 9781409468370 (ebk – PDF)
ISBN 9781409468387 (ebk – ePUB)

MIX Paper from responsible sources FSC® C013985

Printed in the United Kingdom by Henry Ling Limited, at the Dorset Press, Dorchester, DT1 1HD

# Contents

# Preface

I have had a rather broad and mixed audience in mind when writing this book and hope that it will be of relevance to academics, managers, healthcare workers, policy-makers and other practitioners who have an interest in gender and women's and men's health. I also hope that it will be found relevant by students on health and social care courses at both undergraduate and postgraduate levels, including students on qualifying nursing and assistant practitioner programmes. To this end, I have developed the text in an accessible style, determined to write as inclusively as possible making the text suitable for a diverse readership. This is not a highly theoretical book and intentionally so.

With a commitment to interdisciplinarity, I draw on literature from the fields of sociology, management theory, psychology and anthropology. Although cultural theory from anthropology that explores how cultural practices are meaningfully constructed has been useful in challenging claims of universalism associated with gender norms, I do not discuss *foreign* societies in any depth. I draw only on particular examples to develop specific points – usually to problematise dominant or accepted ways of thinking and seeing. This book concentrates on Western industrialised societies, with particular attention given to the UK.

The book has a broad focus, but is mainly concerned with qualitative issues of meaning and understanding of the part played by gender in the experience of health and healthcare work. Quantitative issues of frequencies, variables, correlations and explanations, though considered, are given less priority, as the emphasis in the narrative accounts that make up the volume is interpretative and qualitative. This is because, while statistical analysis may reveal the incidence of phenomena and through standardised descriptors enable systematic comparisons, it has difficulty handling real-world complexity and causality, failing to capture the subtleties and nuances of issues and experience.

The whole field of gender and health is one that is large and still develeoping, so covering all dimensions of this expanding area is not realistic; the contents of the volume is therefore selective reflecting my particular interests and these shaped by a feminist perspective. As much material is omitted as is included and subjectivity is thus a feature of this volume. Through the use of case studies and portraits of individual experience, key issues are highlighted so that these can be followed up in greater depth by those with specific interests in particular areas. The case studies that feature throughout the text have been selected for their potential to contribute to critical debates and unsettle normative understandings and assumptions associated with gender and health.

I draw on recent research as well as seminal literature to examine the ways in which health and being employed as a healthcare worker are impacted by gender, exploring its effects on men as well as women. Working with other people's ideas together with some of my own, I have sought to demonstrate how gender is interwoven into all aspects of the lived experience of health and working for health. Gender is also an important theoretical tool for analysing how power relations between women and men are created and sustained, and this is an underpinning theme of the volume.

## The outline of the book

The concept of health is rich and multi-faceted and, whilst more has been written about illness and disease than about health because of its almost intangible nature, the aspect of human experience that is health is highly valued, even if not much noticed (Downie and Macnaughton, 1998). What is noticed, is the disruption to health through disease and the experience of ill-health and its medical treatment. However, women and men are not only *consumers* of "medicine's miracles" (Pascall, 1997: 180), they are also providers of healthcare labour, both in paid and unpaid roles in private and public settings. Working for health is a source of employment for a wide range of healthcare professionals as well as administrators, managers and a plethora of support workers within an expanding health sector. The curing of disease and the restoration of health comprise the underpinning precepts of modern healthcare practice. The treatment and cure of disease are central to the role of clinical medicine that Porter (1999: 712) claims likes to think of itself as "the most 'beneficent' profession". Health (including ill-health) as experience and work are the two axes along which this volume has been developed. These topics are discussed through the prism of gender that is a significant influence on both the experience and work of health. Much writing on gender and health has highlighted issues of particular concern to women but, as discussion herein demonstrates, men are also gendered health subjects and we are seeing a growing discourse about the 'problem' of men's health and ways to advance male health and wellbeing (Schofield, 2010).

The book begins by introducing in Chapter 1 the key topics explored in the volume, drawing on recent and seminal literature that has informed sociological understanding of the concepts gender, health and work. The concept of gender is developed further in Chapter 2 that highlights the complex and changing constructions of gender from both an historical and material perspective. Gender, as both identity and a set of practices are discussed in ways that draw out characteristics of diversity and fluidity that increasingly shape gender as a significant social category. A discussion of the emergence of masculinities as a separate focus of experience and study closes the chapter.

The different health experiences of women and men are the theme of Chapter 3 which considers female and male patterns of morbidity and mortality as well as notions of 'femaleness' and 'maleness' that shape take up of health services. Disease patterns vary by gender but figures also show areas of gender convergence. In the case of colorectal cancer, for example, the disease accounted for 14 per cent of all cancer diagnoses in men and 12 per cent in women in England in 2008, making this the third most common cause of cancer death for both women and men (ONS, 2011). Figures for death registrations in the UK for the year 2011 (ONS, 2012) show that 44 per cent of male deaths were to those aged 80 and over, compared with 20 per cent in 1974. In contrast a greater percentage of female deaths occurred at ages 80 and over with 62 per cent of all female deaths in 2011 being to women in this age group compared with 40 per cent in 1974.

In Western industrialised societies, women and men have different health careers and this has its roots in gendered ideology associated with the social construction of the family. Specifically the ideological association of femaleness with caring enacted through reproduction and dominant in the private sphere is now embedded in the public sphere with the majority of health and social care work undertaken by women. The topics of the family and the balancing of care and work are the key themes of Chapter 4 that draws particularly on the seminal ideas of Carol Gilligan (1982) that have been so influential in informing the debate about questions of difference related to women's and men's development. Some of these ideas are taken forward in Chapter 5 which traces the politics and practice of work in the healthcare sector from a gendered perspective. The ways in which healthcare roles continue to be gendered are considered against a background of increasing professionalisation and specialisation in healthcare practice that, in recent times, has been characterised by a perceived need for greater credentialism amongst the healthcare workforce. The case studies of nursing, medicine and management frame the discussion.

The significance of technology to all areas of health and healthcare is of increasing importance and this is the topic of Chapter 6. Technology can offer a range of possibilities for improving health, extending life and ameliorating the harmful effects of some harsh medical treatments. However, the design and application of technology for health are not gender neutral and this chapter discusses the ways in which gender influences the use of new technologies in areas such as telecare and reproductive and fertility medicine. Technology is also important for health promotion that, utilising technologies such as screening, aims to draw attention to approaches that both protect and protect health. Chapter 7 explores theoretical ideas and practices that shape contemporary health promotion initiatives through the prism of gender. Discussion of the case studies of gay men's health, breast cancer prevention and coronary heart disease demonstrates that health promotion is an arena of contested social relations, with gender as an important indicator of health beliefs and behaviours.

Chapter 8 has a different tone to earlier chapters which have as an underpinning theme the biomedical model of health that is focused on curing disease. In Chapter 8, however, it is the theme of care that is the focus, with discussion of chronic illness that cannot be cured as the introductory topic. In exploring how gender is implicated in both the experience of incurable disease and its care, the chapter draws on two case studies. The first of these is dementia, now a major global health concern, but particularly so in Western societies. The second is the philosophy and practice of palliative care provided in a range of community and clinical settings. The role of volunteers in hospice-based end-of-life care is highlighted to elucidate how the terrain of care and suffering connected to loss and letting go is still more often associated with the world of women.

Intersectionality that can be understood as a multifaceted lens through which to explore the identity of those excluded from the circles of power through race, gender, class, age, sexuality and disability is the theme of Chapter 9. The chapter's discussion demonstrates that gender is one of a number of social categories that shape the experience of health and working in healthcare roles. It argues that an understanding of the interconnectivity of social differences is necessary for effective healthcare practice, specifically to take account of social inequalities in health.

Chapter 10, as the final chapter in the volume, brings together the main themes with closing summary comments about the way forward for feminism and gender relations. It ends on a positive note, suggesting that feminist activism that foregrounds not just gender but other social differences, will continue to build on its now established collaborative and intersectional stance to be an enduring significant force for social change.

# Chapter 1
# Introduction

Gender and the 'gender order' (Matthews, 1984) have, for some social commentators, begun to be 'unfashionable' topics of enquiry. Gender as a social construct has, in recent times, lost its former conceptual allure to the extent that its ongoing relevance to understanding social organisation and personal behaviour has begun to be questioned, particularly relative to other social categories. Despite this, gender continues to engage many in the academy, and recent work by writers such as Ryle (2012) and Walby (2011) has demonstrated that the gender project, though subject to continuous transformation and interpretation, continues to be integral to the realisation of social democracy achieving its full potential. More specifically, in aligning social democracy with economic democracy and opposing the excesses of capitalism that give rise to inequality, Walby (2011) argues for a stronger articulation of gender within macro-analytical frameworks, citing as an example the full employment of women as necessary for economic growth.

Health status and the experience of working in healthcare roles are both strongly shaped by gender and, although there have been attempts to incorporate gender awareness in both health and employment policies, the significance of gender in these areas continues to be marginalised within public debates and academic discourses that have historically tended towards a gender-neutral perspective. The work of Kuhlmann and Annandale (2010), Gough and Robertson (2010) and Featherstone et al. (2007) has gone some way towards highlighting the ways in which gender materially influences health behaviour and healthcare practice, but this remains an under-theorised area. Focusing more specifically on labour market participation in the health sector, recent empirical work reported by writers such as Karlsen (2012) and Pas et al. (2011) has extended the debate to focus on the importance of gendered norms in culturally shaping clinical careers. Moore's (2009) critique of intersectionality, as a tool to explore how advantage/disadvantage within specific occupations and sectors is reproduced in terms of gender and race, has added to our understanding of how inequality is both complex and layered. Walby et al. (2012), addressing theoretical issues concerning intersectionality, raise important questions about the conceptual and material relationship between multiple inequalities.

These texts are amongst a number that have made a valuable contribution to knowledge about the impact of gender on the experience of health and illness and also on the gendered experience of being employed as a healthcare worker. However, the approach of much recent writing on these topics has been to focus on gender and health or on gender and work rather than taking an integrated perspective on the impact of gender on the wider health domain. This volume offers an integrated discussion of how the experience of health and illness and healthcare work is gendered, to particularly draw out how gender affects the type of health work undertaken by men and women and the rewards they receive for their labour.

This is a complex area, both conceptually and empirically, because of shifting understandings of the ways in which gender is contested and negotiated and the changing environment of healthcare work that in recent years has had to respond to growing demands arising from an ageing population and more sophisticated treatments for a range of conditions. Added to this, health has long been recognised as more than just the absence of disease and, for example, the importance of healthy lifestyles, as part of health promotion initiatives, draws attention to health both as individual responsibility and public good.

The three concepts that provide the underpinning themes of this volume are: gender, health and work. These concepts have been widely debated in the literature from a number of disciplinary perspectives offering a plethora of meanings rendering each beyond simple or straightforward definition. Whilst space does not allow for an in-depth critique of each of these concepts, the principal aim of this chapter is to introduce each in relation to key debates that draw out their contested nature, as a way of setting the scene for the chapters that follow. Gender, as the overarching construct, is explored in more/greater depth in Chapter 2 deserving, as it is, of further scrutiny to uncover its multiple dimensions and historical development.

## Introducing gender

Gender is everywhere around us and is generally taken for granted. We identify a person as a man or a woman and social arrangements of all kinds are organised around this distinction (Connell, 2002; Ryle, 2012). At the level of everyday life, this perceptual and material categorisation that draws on biological sex difference, underpins many practical aspects such as separate toilets in public places for men and women, sporting activities for boys and girls in separate teams and the provision of single-sex schools to name but a few. Gender seems obvious, 'natural' and in terms of the way we relate to one another, reasonably certain. Expectations about the roles men and women have in life, both in the home and in the public sphere, have also continued to be shaped by gender norms. Most childcare is the responsibility of women (Chodorow, 1978) and there are many more men than women in senior business and political positions (Crompton, 2006). Gender roles are the activities a culture assigns to each sex or, put another way, culture takes biological differences and associates them with certain activities. The extent to which these gender divisions are 'natural' has been at the forefront of sociological thinking in this area, particularly since the 1970s and it is sociology that has led the way in distinguishing between sex and gender. Before then, work on sex roles had been marginal to sociology's mainstream concerns (Jackson and Scott, 2002). Other disciplines such as anthropology and psychology have also begun to incorporate gender into their analytical thinking, drawing out its wider cultural and social meanings and this is discussed in more detail in the next chapter.

So, gender as social category has become an established feature of the way we see the world, but is this fixed and mainly (or only) dependent on biological and sexual difference? The idea of sex as part of the 'natural order' renders it as fixed, non-volitional and determined and, as such, *not* socially constructed. Writers such as Connell (2002), Evans (2003), Walby (2011), Ryle (2012) and Carrera et al. (2012) counter the position of biological determinism with their argument that gender is acquired rather than given and that femininity and masculinity are produced through a range of practices and behaviours shaped by dichotomous social expectations of what it means to be male and female. Both women and men are required to engage in different forms of sex-marking behaviour (Frye, 1983) involving, for example, aspects of embodiment and appearance including the choice of clothes and hairstyles and items of adornment such as jewellery and fashion accessories. Whilst such matters are subject to cultural norms and the vagaries of fashion, each person is expected to claim their gender by making clear what sex they are in order to engage in normal social interaction. Efforts aimed at continual gender reinforcement feature across the life-course.

This argument positions gender as socially constructed rather than biologically determined such that our social selves are equally as important as our biological selves in shaping our gender. At a simplistic level, attributes seen as masculine are in opposition to those identified as feminine. Masculine notions of power, authority, objectivity and rationality are contrasted with feminine attributes of sensitivity, nurturing and emotion. However, 'female and male' and 'feminine and masculine' are not necessarily clear and opposite categories. Some people may look and behave in ways that do not neatly fit the labels female/feminine or male/masculine (Holmes, 2009). Bodies as well as affective behaviours also come into play here, particularly given the primacy of bodies in determining gender. An infant being labelled either female or male begins the process of gender socialisation.

Focusing on sexed bodies, Butler (1990) argues that bodies, whilst generally sex-identified at birth through the presence of female/male genitalia, become gendered through the continual performance of gender with this as a process reproducing existing conventions and norms. One thus *becomes* a girl or a boy with this being not simply a fact of nature or, as Holmes (2009: 14) puts it, "gender is not something we naturally *are* but something we learn to *do*". Issues of dress, play, education and bodily adornment are relevant and these aspects are powerful symbols of what it means to be a girl or a boy child. In the West, for example, the colour pink for girls and blue for boys predominates in many areas of material consumer culture. Girls and boys do different subjects at school, often end up in different jobs, and women and men are portrayed differently in the media (Ryle, 2012: 276). It is important to stress, however, that there are significant cross-cultural variations and studies from anthropology which have much to teach us about how gender is produced differently in some non-Western societies. Because anthropologists study biology, culture and society, they are in a unique position to analyse nature (biological predispositions) and nurture (socialisation) as determinants of human behaviour and the cultural construction of male and female identity (Kottak, 2004). Anthropologists have gathered data about similarities and differences involving gender in many cultural contexts uncovering a wide range of diverse gender patterns. In some cultures, for example, a 'third gender' exists and Schmidt (2003) describes how in Samoan Polynesian society some men adopt feminine ways in terms of appearance and social roles and are seen neither as men or women. Two sexes are not sufficient to capture the variety found among human beings, with tension between bodies and identities contributing to gender ambiguity.

Much sociological analysis on gender has its roots in feminist scholarship that has focused attention on men and women as *social* rather than natural categories, challenging the 'naturalness' of differences between men and women and considering ways in which people might resist gender conventions and do things differently (Jackson and Scott, 2002). Central to the contribution of feminist thinking on this topic is the importance placed on exploring the divisions between men and women and the hierarchical relationship between them (Delphy, 1993). Division and hierarchy are the two constitutive elements of gender. The hierarchical relationship, as a form of gender stratification, is characterised by an unequal distribution of rights, resources and power between women and men, with men having the major share. Whilst gender stratification varies across cultures, economies and political systems, a common feature is the distinction between women's reproductive domestic work and men's productive economic labour that reinforces a contrast between men as public and valuable with social status and prestige and women as domestic, home-based, less visible and less valued. The seminal contribution made by feminist scholars to increasing awareness and understanding of the impact of gender on all spheres of social and public life is discussed in more detail in the next chapter. Discussion will include reference to the various political standpoints of particular feminist positions. The distinctions of liberal, radical and socialist feminism are identified in respect of the approach of each to the analysis of gender relations. For the current chapter it is helpful to briefly set out some key points that chart the development of feminist ideas about gender as a political site for thinking about the social environment that shapes women's and men's lives differently.

Brownmiller (1976) and Firestone (1979), writing in the early years of second-wave feminism, argue that women's oppression is primarily due to a universal male control of women's bodies and sexuality, with women's reproductive role at the core of their inferior status. Writers such as Barrett and McIntosh (1982), however, point to the gendering of social relations in both the domestic and public spheres as the cause of women's oppression. They argue that only when the sexual division of labour within the family is eradicated, can women take up an equal economic role with men. Pateman (1988), in her seminal work on contract theory, raises feminist questions about the hidden sexual contract that she contends forms a significant part of the subtext of citizenship, employment and marriage all underpinned by the subjection of women in the private sphere within a system of patriarchy, a system largely controlled by men and operated in their interest. However, she identifies patriarchy as not only familial and located in the private sphere, arguing that patriarchy shapes relations between government, labour and capital in the civil realm.

The concept of patriarchy is taken up and developed by Walby (1986; 1990) in her powerful critique of interrelated patriarchal structures that she sees as reinforcing women's subordination. Her thesis is that patriarchal relations in the home, in the waged labour market, in the operation of the state, in the propensity for male violence against women, in the culture of 'compulsory' heterosexuality and lastly in the cultural values found in art, education, science and religion reproduce structured inequalities and the institutional oppression of women. Walby (1986; 1990) emphasises that this oppression does not derive simply from individual actions, but is built into structural and institutional patterns and policies. Even if men are uncomfortable with this and would like to change it, they still benefit from the overall subordination of women within a male-dominated society in terms of monetary benefits, authority, respect and access to institutional power. Connell (1995: 79) terms this as the 'patriarchal dividend'; he also makes the point that some women participate in the patriarchal dividend by being married to wealthy men. On one level it could be argued that systems that discriminate against women because of their gender have been largely removed through legislation, but as discussion below reveals, dominant gendered expectations about women's and men's roles in society endure and related gender stereotypes continue to be strongly held with negative impacts for women through a range of exclusionary practices.

## Thinking about health

In exploring the question 'what is health?' I will be exploring meanings of health from a variety of perspectives. Drawing on a range of disciplines, the discussion that follows presents contrasting and competing ideas to construct health as individual, familial, social, local and spatial. Health, like gender, is all around us; it is often in the news and is at the centre of public policy in many countries of the West. Whilst most would agree that health is an important issue, there is less agreement on how health is defined and what it means to be healthy. One starting point is the WHO (World Health Organisation) definition: 'Health is a state of complete physical and mental wellbeing and not merely the absence of disease or infirmity' (WHO, 1985). Critics of this definition claim that it is idealistic, utopian and unrealistic, particularly given the enormous disparity in terms of wealth and resources both between and within countries across the globe. And, though there is certainly a debate to be had about the utility of the WHO definition, it does establish that health is multi-dimensional and holistic encompassing physical, emotional, psychological, social and mental aspects. Warwick-Booth et al. (2012) augment this holistic stance on defining health arguing that health involves a range of subjectivities and experiences that are socially, historically and culturally located. As an example, the link between poverty and poor health in contemporary society has been well evidenced such that Graham (2009: 1) contends that: "the opportunity to live a long and healthy life remains profoundly unequal". However, the association between income and mortality, widely accepted today, may be a more recent phenomenon. Bengtsson and van Poppel (2011), analysing mortality data from locations across Europe and North America up to the first part of the twentieth century, argue for a reconsideration of the causal link between income and mortality. Whatever the causal factors, the social distribution of health continues to exercise policy-makers and those working on the frontline delivering a range of healthcare services (Sheaff, 2005).

Further recent thinking has directed attention to other characterisations of health such as quality of life, lifestyle choices and health consumerism positioning health as something that can be chosen and performed and also as a commodity that can be bought and sold like any other in the market place. Health means different things to different people and, with the emergence of more pluralistic notions of 'being healthy', health is no longer dominated by more medical and scientific explanations. Taking exercise, eating fresh unprocessed food, watching one's weight, keeping fit and actively participating in society are all now seen as indicators of health. In former times it was the absence of illness that was seen as the primary health indicator. Concepts of health are changing and being and remaining healthy is a core activity within our society. However, health depends not only on what goes on inside our bodies, but also on the conditions under which we live and work. Individual susceptibilities may play a part, but many of the preconditions for health are beyond the control of any but the privileged few. Health is thus highly political and the politics of health are discussed in Chapter 7 which considers health promotion as a positive concept emphasising social and personal resources of all kinds as well as physical and mental capabilities.

Health is culturally produced with its meaning varying considerably from society to society and from one historical period to another. The cultural construction of health has long been the concern of anthropology that has contributed much to our understanding of health as social construction and cultural practice through production of detailed ethnographies of many types of societies, both indigenous and developed. Medical anthropology has become a thriving branch of the discipline shedding light on the values of indigenous methods in coping with ill-health and on the ways that various human populations respond to ageing and bodily deterioration (Hendry, 2008: 296). Anthropologists have also had an important contribution to make to world health programmes, advising about potential cultural sensitivities to certain medical approaches in local contexts.

Notions of health and illness drawn from ethnographic studies are useful in offering alternative ways of thinking about what it means to be 'well' and what it means to be 'ill'. Davis (2000), for example, writing about illness and therapy among the Tabwa of Central Africa, reports that when asked to define the condition of health, people described it as a state in which one feels *nothing* and one just goes about ordinary life as usual. This might well resonate with many of us in the West when asked to consider the same question. Health has an invisible and intangible quality and is not something on which we routinely focus, at least not on a day-to-day basis. Davis (2000: 65) comments further that: "a healthy body has a well-balanced relation to its environment, external and internal". 'Wellness' is signified through whole bodily and mental balance as a desired external and inner state of harmony. In health, forces of a potentially pathological nature are kept in abeyance to maintain an overall balance. In illness the situation is reversed with the balance of well-functioning organs thrown into a state of disorder resulting in the breakdown of bodily integrity. Illness, though in opposition to health, is nevertheless accepted as a necessity leading to death as part of the cycle of life. Davis (2000) reports the words of a Tabwa man receiving treatment for tuberculosis; when Davis offered reassurance the man responded with a question: "have you ever seen a thing which did not die?" Despite an innate acceptance of death as natural, tribal societies, in effect, maintain individual and group health by emphasising prevention of morbidity rather than treatment of disease (Baer et al., 2003). The emphasis on *prevention* has now also become a pivotal aspect of much health promotion in many countries of the West (see Chapter 7).

Ideas about health change, but so also does health itself. HIV/AIDS and significant levels of drug addiction are two diseases of the modern age present in both developed and less developed societies. These are diseases of the global system, affecting people of every age, race, class, ethnicity, gender and sexual orientation. The sudden appearance of AIDS in the early 1980s was unexpected and, in the Western context, challenged the notion that mortality from infectious disease was a thing of the past. AIDS has revealed itself as a disease of social relationship – not merely a social disease (Baer et al., 2003: 230) and, with its rapid spread the term *epidemic* was thrust back into popular language invoking notions of high-risk personal behaviour and the threat to health from some intimate encounters. The health status associated with these conditions is socially constructed as deviant and subject to social opprobrium and public disparagement evoking a range of responses from tolerance through to empathy and disgust (Campbell and Ettorre, 2011). In the case of AIDS, there is the added stigma that those suffering with the disease are being punished for their deviant behaviour leading Baer et al. (2003: 238) to comment that: "the social damages of stigmatization are equal to if not more painful than the medical consequences of the disease". The stigma impact of AIDS has only been partially mitigated by the widespread appearance of the disease among some receiving blood transfusions; their position, as one without personal guilt, is attributed victim status.

Other changes in health identified by Taylor and Bury (2007) are an ageing population, better housing, smaller family sizes, increased standards of living, female emancipation and shifts from manual to knowledge-based occupations as shaping overall improvements in health in the West. Malnutrition, as a disease of poverty, has now in affluent societies been overtaken by obesity, a disease of plenty as a major health issue, particularly amongst disadvantaged groups in those societies. Whilst the physical stress associated with hard manual labour is in decline, the psychological stress connected to fast-paced demanding service sector and knowledge-based work is on the increase. Added to this, wider access to information from the internet and the media about health and disease has transformed relationships within healthcare – no longer are doctors seen as the ultimate or only authority, a position that was the case for long periods in the past (Kellehear, 2007). Health and healthcare are now subject to negotiation and the notion of *professional expertise* amongst a range of healthcare workers has been challenged by patients exploring for themselves information about diseases and treatments. Challenges to traditional systems of medical power and knowledge give rise to forms of resistance such as seeking a second diagnostic opinion, use of alternative therapies or the refusal to take medical advice.

The boundary between expert and lay knowledge is shifting and increasingly patients are becoming experts in their own disease, contributing to research and collaborating with healthcare professionals on clinical education programmes. Patients' views are also now widely sought about a range of issues connected to the management and delivery of healthcare (Martin, 2007). This change has been termed by some as *patient power* that is integral to the democratisation of healthcare seen by Prior (2003) as being more customer-sensitive and based on a partnership model developed through participation mechanisms such as patient panels and advisory groups. The change is also a feature of a growth in the market-based model of health where patients are notionally positioned as consumers. It could be argued that 'patients as customers' contribute to an empowerment model of health that encourages active navigation of the health system. This model is now a feature of much health service provision in many countries of the West. However, the re-positioning of the patient as empowered and *responsibilised* consumer of health through consultation and knowledge processes (Lupton, 2002), masks the blurred boundaries between empowerment and compliance arising from lay knowledge that remains a contested domain of expertise (Allsop et al., 2004; Harris et al., 2010). This patient/expert partnership approach is mirrored in much healthcare delivery by multi-professional teams comprising a range of specialties such as physiotherapists, nurses, doctors, occupational therapists and radiographers working together to deliver healthcare to the individual patient. Relationships between patients and healthcare professionals are being redefined with reduced emphasis on hierarchies as a function of the biomedical model and more attention now being given to health as a collaborative process (Martin and Finn, 2011).

Health is not a straightforward concept. It involves minimising disease and maximising physical, psychological and social wellbeing. Health levels are affected by biomedical advances of all kinds including technological advances and the development of drug therapies for a whole range of conditions. We have come to view medical systems primarily in terms of what they do – that is, in terms of the therapeutic and health-improving action they may make possible. We use the language of health solutions and health is now big business, for drug companies, for healthcare organisations and for clinicians, many of whom, in the role of consultant physicians, are very highly paid with income from both National Health Service (NHS) work and private practice. Whilst the pursuit of finding cures for life-limiting conditions such as cancer and heart disease continues and progresses at a significant rate, the drive to extend life is served in many cases by the possibility that biological life *can* be sustained through the use of sophisticated (and often technologically complex) surgical interventions. The quantity versus quality of life debate and the role of medical ethics in determining what *should* be done in the best interests of patients is eloquently taken up by Schneiderman and Jecker (2011). They argue for more realistic expectations in medicine and a more humane view of health and wellbeing in the face of life-limiting illness. These issues will be discussed in Chapter 6, but are very much part of current health debates as well as part of how we see health and thus pertinent to this opening chapter.

Healthy communities and localities bring a spatial and environmental emphasis to the meaning of health. The social circumstances in which people live contribute to the health of individuals and families and there is growing recognition that the planning and design of neighbourhoods can influence the health of people living in them. Housing and the wider built local environment that includes shops, libraries, parks and leisure facilities help to shape healthy communities. Poor housing, with people living in damp, noisy and cramped conditions can influence mental as well as physical health. Mental health does not just mean the absence of a specific disorder but is wider including how people handle stress and how people see themselves and their lives. The lack of safe outside space for children to play is another factor that can add to the frustration of children and families. It can also lead to children developing behavioural problems.

Schools also influence health with many making their sports facilities available to the local community in the evenings and at weekends. The work of school nurses contributes to health education programmes that focus on drugs, contraception and HIV/AIDS. Immunisation and vaccination programmes are also run in schools. The idea that schools should be a place where children develop healthy bodies as well as attain academically has long been a feature of education provision. The attention given to the provision of nutritious food in schools to reinforce healthier eating patterns is one example of the ways in which schools intervene to improve the health of their pupils; breakfast clubs are another. Workplaces, too, impact on health and, despite the growth of health and safety legislation, workplaces can negatively impact on the health of those who work in them.

There are many ways to think about health and discussion above has pointed to the social and local, as well as to the individual nature of health. The experience of health is also intensely personal and the complex life conditions of women and men bring gender to the heart of health. Kuhlmann and Annandale (2010) argue that gender is strongly associated with health status and exerts a significant influence upon both help-seeking behaviour and the delivery of healthcare. Social patterning of health and healthcare, they argue, is gendered and issues connected to women's and men's health have now begun to be the concern of policy-makers, though usually in terms of women's and men's illnesses rather than in relation to wellbeing. Although gender-sensitive healthcare has its roots in feminist activism, specifically as action to counter the systematic devaluation of women, gender awareness in health is now seen to involve men's health thus expanding the concept of gender beyond women's issues (Broom and Tovey, 2009). This is part of the wider concept of gender mainstreaming of approaches to the design, implementation and monitoring of public services of all kinds including the health sector. The ultimate aim is the achievement of gender equality. Gender relations in health that includes the growing body of knowledge from studies on masculinities, is discussed in Chapter 3 that considers men's and women's health in relation to gender specific diseases such as testicular and breast cancer and the medicalisation of women's reproductive capacities across the life-course.

## Conceptualising work and the issue of gender

As with gender and health, the concept of work has been the subject of extensive sociological enquiry and there now exists a highly developed literature on all aspects of work and society. Work as concept and practice is diverse and definitions and categories from a number of disciplines have developed and include: paid and voluntary work; public/private sector work; part and full-time work; service work; manufacturing work; unionised and non-unionised work; professional and unskilled work and employed and self-employed work arrangements. Drawing mainly on ideas from sociology, further categories have the labels 'women's work' (usually referring to low status tasks such as cleaning and care work and shop work), 'dirty work' such as refuse collection and street cleaning and manual/physical work that, however essential or skilled, is seen as undignified and inferior to intellectual or professional work (Edgell, 2006). The stigma associated with certain types of work, particularly when undertaken by marginal groups, persists as integral to the widely accepted social hierarchy of occupational structures in today's Western society.

Different types of work and employment arrangements are the subjects of extensive critical focus and there is now a separate corpus of literature on the sociology of management, human resources, industrial relations, business theory and organisations. These varying features of work incorporate different elements of the employment relationship and point to a complex conceptual terrain for work sociologists to investigate. The way we view work is shaped by our social position in terms of class, gender, ethnicity and age and for most people work takes up a substantial proportion of their lives and is a source of status and value, as well as the means by which the activities and responsibilities of life are financed. Indeed, the economic necessity to work, termed by some as 'working to live', contributes to the moral necessity and obligation to work characterised as both private and public good. Noon and Blyton (2007) add that in many societies in the West and in Asia and Africa, the model of 'working to consume', both commodities and services, has taken hold as the prime motivation to work, with this both fuelling and fuelled by spiralling global consumption.

The dominant view of work as formal paid employment is a product of the emergence of Western industrial capitalist society in the nineteenth and twentieth centuries. In particular, the rise of manufacturing and the factory system gave rise to a demarcation between home and work so that increasingly those in employment *went out* to a place of work. Before then in the pre-industrial era, women's and men's work tasks overlapped and family units were the sites of production in both town and country, based primarily on a domestic system of manufacture at home and in small workshops (Rendall, 1990). Industrial development transformed the process of production, making it possible to produce on a large scale what had formerly been produced by the household. There were exceptions to this home-based model and, for example, work in the mills and factories, in shipbuilding and in the mines, though small-scale by later standards, did involve an organised labour process requiring workers to travel to these centres of work (Grint, 2005). Clearly, work has centuries of earlier history but the age of early capitalism saw a shift from work as a way of life, with an emphasis on social/familial organisation of work tasks to work as an end in itself necessary to finance the activities of life, increasingly shaped by economic market forces.

Work can be enjoyable and satisfying, and a way of fulfilling individual potential. It can also be mundane (a form of wage slavery), damaging to health and, in some settings, subject to extreme forms of control and regulation, with this as one form of what Noon and Blyton (2007: 67) term 'disciplined compliance'. Grint (2005) identifies the ambiguous nature of work as important to the wider understanding of work in both historical and contemporary contexts. Mooney (2004: 18) extends this perspective arguing that: "work is both a source of inequality and a reflection of wider social divisions within society". Most texts on work have confined their attention to work as paid employment that has long been understood to contribute to individual identity, particularly masculine identity, with the ideology of the male breadwinner still the focus of contemporary critiques of the sociology of work (Mooney, 2004; Edwards and Wajcman, 2005; Warren, 2007). Despite this, debates amongst late modern theorists have begun to surface about the extent of work's significance as a source of identity and social affiliation, with identity needs seen as increasingly fulfilled in multiple other realms (Foster, 2012). Although conscious reflection on how work shapes identity revolves primarily around individualised values, it does appear to be culturally encouraged. The connection between *who you are* and *what you do* (in terms of work) is taken up by Howard and Welbourn (2004) who report on the spiritual properties of work that, they argue, are an important element in people's sense of meaning and purpose, contributing significantly to their sense of self in the world.

The concept of work is thus multi-dimensional and, though not subject to essentialist or universalistic definitions, the association of work with paid employment continues to dominate, particularly in relation to social policy and this despite current political rhetoric in the UK of the value of volunteering as part of the 'big society' model. In recent times, however, work as paid labour, has undergone significant transformation, particularly in Western societies that have seen a decrease in manufacturing, the disappearance of a 'job for life', a huge increase in women's employment often in the service sector and, with the onset of the internet, a rise in home and flexible working (Bolton and Houlihan, 2009). A further change has been the growth of the voluntary sector that, heavily charity-based, is characterised by a variety of organisations from large professional bureaucracies to small neighbourhood-based community groups (Newman and Mooney, 2004). The voluntary sector provides paid employment of all kinds together with opportunities for people to engage in different forms of voluntary work. In recent times there has been increased attention paid to the work of volunteers and the promotion of the idea of an active civil society by successive UK governments has led to the professionalisation of some voluntary work as the product of a partnership between the voluntary sector, government and business (Watts, 2012).

The historical development of work as commodified paid labour discussed above, with the workplace as separate and distinct from the home, has led within sociological theory to the doctrine of separate spheres and this has changed fundamentally the way people think about work. Work became something done outside the home for pay and mainly by men, leading to the emergence of men having sole-provider status and this seen as a prime masculine trait (Faludi, 1991). The work undertaken at home mainly by women for no pay became largely invisible, devalued and not seen as work. The primacy of men in paid work roles led to them being paid a *family wage* necessary to sustain all members of the family and this reflected the ideology of the male breadwinner and endorsed by protective labour legislation (Ryle, 2012). This model provided justification for paying women less, as their wage was perceived as supplementary to that of their husbands. The idea of a wage is thus not a gender-neutral concept and has been used to both marginalise women's earning power and maintain their position of dependency on men. The male breadwinner model does not take account of women supporting themselves and their families without the contribution of a male partner. For middle-class women the opportunity for paid work was only possible until they married, with this custom observed well into the twentieth century (Comer, 1974).

The gender wage gap is important because it remains a significant determinant of inequality between women and men. With less money, women have less power in family settings and more generally have access to fewer resources. A major part of the gender pay gap is accounted for by gendered job segregation due to women and men working in different occupations. Put simply, masculinised jobs pay more (Magnusson, 2010) and Alvesson and Due Billing (1997) outline how, in many industries after the onset of capitalism, work was designed according to one or other gender. This, they argue, was also the case in respect of the fast developing public services. By designating jobs as women's work, it was possible to employ women more cheaply than men because of the lower social value already placed on their labour.

Whilst the importance of work to men's lives is rarely questioned and, for many, is central to their core identity, this is not seen to apply to women in the same way, due mainly to the traditional sexual division of labour that Morris (1999) characterises as being ideologically central to the work–family–welfare nexus. The increase of female employment both during and after the Second World War, a greater number of women entering higher education and the impact of feminism have challenged traditional sex roles as part of the struggle for women's liberation. Feminism, the mobilising agent for women's liberation, has always been concerned about women's participation or non-participation in paid employment and early radical feminist activism was just as focused on women's right to work and be paid equally to men as it was on the cause of suffrage (Freedman, 2001).

It is these issues that have been at the forefront of feminist debates about the nature of work, how it is valued and the position of women in the labour market, particularly how they negotiate the demands of paid work with those of family work. Being reproductively female or male plays a determining role in differential access to the labour market, occupational location, workplace conditions and rates of pay. Exposing this has been at the heart of the feminist project. Thus feminist critiques of classical sociological accounts of work and employment have sought to uncover their generally gender-neutral focus, specifically to illuminate women's peripheral position in the labour process as well as their 'hidden' role in reproducing the family, with Oakley (1974) pressing for recognition of women's domestic work as having economic as well as social value. Feminist writers such as Evans (2003) and Saul (2003), for example, argue that women's unequal access to jobs that carry organisational power and women's concentration in low-paid work are primarily a gender issue due to the continuing domestic pattern whereby women perform the greater share of household work and childcare.

The contemporary gendered division of labour is the result of a long historical process with enduring cultural conceptions about the roles women and men are expected to perform (Alvesson and Due Billing, 1997). My own research that explored the position of women in professional construction roles (see Watts, 2007a; 2009) found that opportunities for women to advance their careers were significantly restricted once they became mothers. This impact has been termed by Magnusson (2010) as the motherhood penalty. Women in my study, in the role of highly skilled civil engineers, were seen and treated differently by both male and female colleagues once they had had children, particularly in relation to their flexibility and availability in the highly competitive construction industry. For these women, a crucial issue was having a positive work/life balance, an issue that has come to be seen as part of a new politics of quality of life affecting both women and men (Christie and Jacobs, 2000). The extent to which the growth of paid female employment and concerns about work/life balance are inter-related is the subject of ongoing debate. Lewis (2002) argues that the rapid rise in female employment is changing attitudes to traditional role expectations (both within and outside the home) resulting in the emergence of de-gendered roles, particularly amongst middle-class couples.

The above critique presents a brief summary of ideas about the history, meaning and gendered nature of work as an introduction to later chapters that consider particular aspects of the gendering of some healthcare roles. Gender issues at work are often subtle, difficult to address and sometimes interwoven with other inequalities such as race, age and disability. This is a complex area and differentiating types of gender issues is useful in helping to develop understanding of gender at work as dynamic and layered. DeLaat (1999: 2), who has written extensively about gender in the workplace, has identified a range of workplace gender issues that she classifies into five main categories. The first is *gender stereotyping*, for example, 'men don't become midwives'. The second is *gender discrimination in compensation, promotion and benefits* that a number of commentators have termed as glass ceiling issues. The third concerns *career development and mentoring* and the fourth is *balancing work and family responsibilities*, that is, child and elder care, dual career couples and pregnancy issues. The last of the five categories is *sexual harassment* that encompasses a wide range of behaviours and, though predominantly so, does not refer only to the harassment of women by men. Unwanted sexual attention of any kind constitutes sexual harassment (Stanko, 1988) and has the effect of lowering a victim's self-confidence and reducing their motivation and productivity. Some of these gender issues will come under scrutiny later in the volume through discussion of case study material and it is important here in this opening chapter to outline their taxonomy to aid understanding of what can seem highly theoretical and abstract notions.

In summary, a pattern of gender-differentiated work experiences, occupations and rewards continues today and Grint (2005) briefly outlines some of the key features of the current 'work landscape' from a gender perspective. Women are paid less than men, have fewer opportunities for promotion, are usually found in unskilled or semi-skilled service jobs, are more likely to work part-time and tend to combine paid employment with unpaid domestic family care work. They are, however, less likely than men to be unemployed and are now found in more executive and senior management roles than was the case in earlier times, though they remain significantly under-represented at all levels of the science and engineering sector. In terms of occupational involvement women play a dominant role within social services, health and service sectors, teaching and retail, while men predominate in technical fields, defence and transport industries and all types of senior management.

Although this summary provides a very generalised picture of gendered aspects of the labour market, it is helpful in highlighting some of the features of disadvantage that accrue to women and also some of the structural changes that are occurring and impacting on the experience of work for both women and men. Although contemporary debates about work now increasingly engage with issues such as work/life balance, flexible working, capital restructuring and the challenges of globalisation, gender continues to be a prominent and often contentious feature of the employment relationship, with growing political rhetoric directed towards its consideration.

## Conclusion

A number of analyses of gender have been developed, some emphasising the power difference between men and women (particularly the economic basis of male power), while others have stressed the differences between men and women highlighted in the sex/gender system. Whatever the approach, gender is now understood not only as a set of attributes connected to individuals, but as a wider set of meanings and discourses. Feminist concerns with power, plurality and diversity and the dismantling of oppositional categories such as those used to *define* women and men, have been extended to other domains beyond sociology to position gender at the centre of understanding about all kinds of lived experience. Gender comprises a spectrum of meaning beyond simple classification of female and male categories. The work we do, the income we earn, expectations about caring roles specifically *who* cares, physical and mental health and access to health services all involve gendered processes. The health needs of women and men are not the same and a gender sensitive approach to the ways in which services are provided is some way from being fully realised.

The intricacies of gender are many and complex and, though much research has found gender to be of pivotal importance to understanding the experience of health and being employed in the workplace (in healthcare roles and in the wider labour market), the wide-ranging significance of gender is still not taken sufficiently into account when considering health and employment policies and practice. The situation, however, is changing though the slow speed of that change continues, giving rise to ongoing academic and political debates about what further can be done to incorporate gender awareness alongside issues of race and class to improve health outcomes for all and achieve greater gender equality in the workplace. The gender project is multi-faceted and changing and some might claim that it has had its day. I do not subscribe to that view and a key aim of this book is to contribute ideas and understanding about the components and dynamics of gender, specifically to identify how these affect the experience of health and healthcare work.

In this chapter readers have been introduced to the concepts of gender, health and work in a way that situates them within sociological enquiry. Whilst other disciplines have been shown to contribute understanding of their meaning, sociology remains central to the interpretation of ideas presented in the chapters that follow. In the next chapter ideas about gender as socially constructed are developed from both a historical and material perspective. Gender, as a significant social category and critical analytical site, is subject to contradictions, changing mores and diversity. Gender, as a fluid concept, is thus the underpinning theme of Chapter 2.

# Chapter 2
# Constructing and Deconstructing Gender

## Introduction

This chapter explores the social construction of gender highlighting the complexity of this concept from both an historical and material perspective. A key aim of the chapter is to introduce readers to the ongoing debates and contradictions of gender as a significant social category, particularly the emergence of masculinities as a separate focus of experience and study. An important feature of this debate is the issue of diversity that can so easily be lost in the dominant, often polarised discourse about what it means to be a woman or a man. Much of this discourse continues to be shaped by the notion of sex identity established within a binary system of male and female and, because sex and gender are so often conflated, the biological inevitability of the sex organs becomes associated with assigned social roles related to gender (Gottlieb, 2002). At a fundamental biological level, it can be argued that female and male, as essential embodiment, can be defined in terms of biological reproductive functionality. Even at this level, however, sex definition can be problematic; does the girl/woman, who lives as female, but does not possess a womb forfeit the right to claim femaleness? Similarly in relation to maleness, does a man who is unable to produce sperm abandon an identity as a man, because his 'real' masculinity may be undermined? These kinds of questions serve to illustrate how sex and gender are interwoven both conceptually and as lived experience.

Disentangling the concepts sex and gender, that involves problematising assumed progress from biology to the social, from male to masculinity and from female to femininity, has been central to the feminist project which has identified gender as the foundation of a profoundly unequal social world (Evans, 2003). Sex and gender are unstable categories and human sexual identity is complex and, for some, a source of ambivalence, not least because femininity and masculinity are not *natural* but *acquired*. Tying feminine and masculine 'norms' to modes of reproduction and production is also central to the construction of heterosexuality that continues to shape normative understandings of the family, idealised and located in the private sphere, the subject of much scrutiny by feminist scholars. Questioning *traditional* family forms and their dominant relations of power based on men's productive and women's reproductive work has been a major focus for feminists of all political persuasions and especially so for socialist feminists. The feminist thesis is that as differences between women and men are socially constructed they can be changed and constraining women to reproductive roles (mainly within the family) is a feature, not of a mature society but of a backward-looking one (Barrett and McIntosh, 1982). Defining gender sociologically through understanding how femininity and masculinity have been socially constructed in a world of binary oppositions has enormous implications, both theoretically and experientially (Chancer and Watkins, 2006). Whilst much of this debate would now be familiar to most of us, these kinds of arguments highly publicised in the 1960s, 70s and 80s, were powerful in both their vehemence and their undisguised attack on patriarchal systems seen as being at the root of women's oppression. The development of these ideas is discussed below mainly in the context of second-wave feminism that heralded a new period of feminist collective political activism (Pilcher and Whelan, 2004: 144).

## Gender and feminism – historical reflections and theoretical directions

Sociology, more than any other discipline, has had a pivotal role to play in the development of ideas about gender. In its early beginnings, sociology was largely the domain of white, mainly European, upper-class men (Ryle, 2012) whose focus was principally on explaining social problems arising from industrialisation and capitalism with the assumption that men's and women's experiences of the world were more or less the same. Women were not included in research and, neither, were they seen as having anything significant or different to contribute to understanding the social world. This gender-blind stance of sociology in its early years had the effect of reinforcing the existing gender order and placing women beyond a sociological theoretical gaze. So, although the ideas of thinkers such as Mary Wollstonecraft, writing in Britain in 1792, set down a marker for later activism aimed at gaining legislative change towards gender equality in relation to property ownership, employment rights and divorce rights, they had little influence on wider theorising on gender in the development of early sociological thinking. One of the first challenges to this position came from Dorothy Smith (1974) with her pioneering critique of the androcentric assumptions underpinning mainstream sociology. She argued for ways in which sociology could be reconfigured from women's perspective with this view eventually becoming known as the feminist standpoint.

Gender, as an analytic category, was similarly absent in the early work of anthropologists mainly because anthropology was also almost exclusively a male activity underpinned by an empirical positivist detached approach to data collection and analysis. However, it was the pioneering work of American female anthropologist, Margaret Mead that drew attention to the binary model of gender construction. Mead's (1935) now seminal ethnography of the indigenous peoples of Papua New Guinea pointed to polarity as an intrinsic feature of gender construction with the essentialist approach of aligning women with nature and men with culture and reason. This theme was later taken up by another American anthropologist, Sherry Ortner (1974) who argued that all societies recognise and make a distinction between culture and the natural world, with culture seen as superior in its attempts to control and transcend nature. So prior to the women's movement becoming fully established in the 1970s and 1980s in the countries of the West, we can trace the stirrings of feminist theory starting to gain currency in the social science academy. Such stirrings also began to appear in psychology and the work of Phyllis Chesler (1972) that explored women's treatment for mental health problems, revealed how male clinicians consistently defined women's reality for them based on an assumption of women's inadequacies rather than those of society. This was powerful stuff and drew on the feminist model of patriarchy that was beginning to emerge as a critical analytical feature of gender theory.

In historical terms the period of first-wave feminism that began to raise awareness about women's lack of civil and employment rights, goes back to the nineteenth century and builds on ideas and concerns of earlier writers such as Wollstonecraft. The focus of the feminist movement at this time was very much centred on women's emancipation and entry into the 'public' realm in terms of access to education and entry into the professions. This early feminism, led mainly by middle-class women and characterised as 'equal rights' feminism, developed a campaigning stance on a wide range of issues of concern to women including improving the legal rights of married women (Banks, 1981). By the beginning of the twentieth century, however, the dominant focus of feminist activism was the issue of the vote and, although brought together in a common cause, divisions between feminist groups began to emerge, split mainly over the various tactics to be used to achieve this goal.

Much has been written about the women's suffrage movement in relation to its high profile leaders and the strategies used to achieve change. For the purpose of this discussion a useful point made by Banks (1981) highlights how a necessary but expedient unity in the movement was short-lived and how after the vote had been achieved, new feminist demands centring on the role of women in the home and their roles as mothers, gave rise to disaffection on the part of 'equal rights' feminists who wanted women to broaden their horizons beyond the home. Getting the vote was only the beginning and not the end of the struggle for gender equality. At the root of the ideological dissonance that began to engulf feminist politics at this time is the vexed question of whether feminist action should focus on women as equal to or different from men. Freedman (2001: 8) cites this as "the perennial feminist problematic" that she argues calls for recognition that feminism is not one unitary concept. Viewing the women's movement in terms of *feminisms* may thus be more appropriate given the different political and social standpoints taken by feminist theorists and activists. That aside, the divergence of the *two feminisms* in the 1920s and 30s marks the transition from first-wave feminist activism to second-wave feminism that has been so influential in calling attention to the social construction of gender.

The second-wave feminist movement, that took hold in the 1960s in the global North, can be seen as part of a larger global social movement that included colonial liberation movements in the developing world and civil rights and student activism in America (Ryle, 2012). Locating second-wave feminism within wider social activism is important in helping to understand that feminism was just one of a number of ideological 'freedom'-type movements emerging in the post-war period, each with its own language, ideas, history and practice. The boundaries of each, however, were less distinct and the connections between different social movements in terms of cross-fertilisation of ideas and tactics were influential, not least in engendering a sense of wider social solidarity between disadvantaged groups. The politics of identity(ies) and feminism were entangled across a continuum of disadvantage involving increasingly complex configurations.

For this volume the focus on second-wave feminism is directed towards uncovering its important contribution to the theorisation of gender, with this seen by some as principally a political project (Barrett and McIntosh, 1982). Personal and sexual politics lie at the centre of theoretical debates about the social position of women and men and, while in the early phase of second-wave feminism the lens was very sharply directed at the unequal social position of women, this gradually gave way to a wider focus on difference and inequality within both genders. This issue of diversity is considered below in more detail and is briefly referred to here to highlight aspects of evolutionary development of second-wave feminist thinking that has come to incorporate a range of theoretical positions. This leads us to consider how and why second-wave feminism, as a diffuse social movement, had the critical exploration of gender as a primary goal. To be clear, as with all social movements, no single geographically-located group or one organisation was leading the way in setting this agenda. In local communities, in colleges and in special interest groups, through consciousness-raising sessions, women were finding connections between their personal lives and the politics of gender. In many ways this was a 'bottom up' movement with groups of women meeting in people's homes, church halls and in workplace settings to discuss their experiences of sexual harassment, domestic violence, reproductive rights, pornography and employment rights, with the debate fuelled by a strong sense of the injustice of existing circumstances for women (Segal, 1999).

As women were beginning to question and break free from their 'biological fate', the relevance of gender in explaining both the social construction of femininity and the maintenance of men's power and privileges relative to women, became heightened. Gender, as the term for all the culturally acquired attributes for becoming a woman (and a man), was adopted, interrogated and theorised by feminists, intent on using gender theory to 'nail' the sex/gender distinction. However, because as Segal (1999) points out, 'man' was the linguistic universal norm for humanity, it was women who were overwhelmingly marked out by gender and categorised as gendered beings. It would be many years before men were fully incorporated into the gender frame, with masculinities eventually emerging as a separate area of study in its own right and this is discussed later in the current chapter.

The many strands of feminism have been the subject of much comment in the literature and I do not propose here to document the detail of how particular feminist standpoints have developed. Instead, I think it is more useful for the purposes of this volume to briefly identify some of the key feminist thinkers across a number of traditions, highlighting their particular contribution to gender theory development. Some might argue that it was Betty Friedan who began to uncover the reality of gender in the every day lives of women when in the late 1950s she set about talking to women about themselves, about their lives as wives and mothers living in suburban settings in the US. What she found and later recounted in *The Feminine Mystique* (Friedan, 1963) was groundbreaking at the time. Supposedly happy and fulfilled in their home-making roles, women told a different story recounting feelings of disappointment, lack of fulfilment and in some cases, despair over the relentless drudgery of being at home. This issue, characterised by Friedan as "the problem with no name", was difficult to own up to because of the association of home-making with womanhood and femininity. Although Friedan's project was more one of journalistic discovery than a piece of methodologically rigorous research and thus having been the subject of considerable criticism, it was and remains seminal because of its focus on women's voices telling women's stories. Women's experiences were placed centre stage and this was a radical departure from former times. The capturing of how women felt trapped and defined by gender difference, specifically by their nurturant domestic attributes, is a powerful critique of how gender at that time was played out and routinely reproduced in many families. Its middle-class and mono-cultural lens is a shortcoming, but prior to this, knowledge about women's lives was constructed only by men and in that sense, in the later words of Eva Figes (1970: 12), women could be seen as "man-made".

Betty Friedan had described the reality of [some] women's lives and it was left to other, often radical, feminist writers to explain it. Kate Millett (1970), in her fierce and uncompromising text *Sexual Politics,* vigorously took up this challenge delivering a powerful critique of the ways in which men through history had prioritised male self-interest in the making of knowledge. Exploring a range of literary genres for her primary sources of evidence, Millett specifically focused on the role of patriarchy in sexual relations arguing that these were essentially relations of dominance with men as the rulers and women as the ruled. As Spender (1985) comments, Millett had made men the enemy. This was controversial and divisive, with some feminists taking the view that, such radical ideas which did not take into account the characteristics of individual men and fostered the homogenisation of men as material and symbolic category, would only heighten tensions between the sexes and were unlikely to advance the cause of women. Whilst the controversy over Millett's thesis still continues, the contribution it has made to theorising patriarchy and highlighting the inevitable power relations of the gender order is very significant and remains a reference point for contemporary writing in this area.

The term 'the personal is political', though now a rather tired mantra, was held by some to encapsulate the essence of feminism and is still regularly invoked to signal that all personal experience is shaped by exterior political forces. The term, first used by Robin Morgan (1970), referred to a new way of seeing and reporting on the world, through the lens of personal experience rather than adopting objective authoritative male-defined credentials. Its message that encourages women to see how inequality affects them, that problems they face are not individual but collective, points to the possibility that these problems can have political solutions. This new way of seeing opened up possibilities for women to explain and represent their lives as historically rooted in patriarchy but not defeated by it, enabling them to produce with confidence their own meanings and cultural forms without reference to men. In the early 1990s when I was embarking on my own personal feminist journey these ideas were inspirational and gave me an alternative framework with which to consider my life, both past and present.

Because a key theme of this volume is work and the gendered relations of employment (specifically in the healthcare sector), the ideas of Juliett Mitchell who focused her analysis on women in the workplace provide valuable insights. Her aim was to explain the exploitation of women in the workforce and her theoretical contribution to gender theory was to link their position in the labour market to women's role in the family. This has now become an accepted theoretical focus of analysis as elucidated by Sylvia Walby and others, but at the beginning of the 1970s, these ideas were radical. Mitchell's (1971) volume *Women's Estate* set out the material conditions of women's role in the home providing services to spouse and children that constrained their entry to the workplace. The four structures identified by Mitchell that would have to be reformed to emancipate women as paid workers were: production, reproduction, sexuality and the care and socialisation of children. These issues continue to be debated today more than 40 years on and remain as sites for exploration and change.

Evolving discourses of feminist thought eventually found their way into the academy and in the late 1980s and early 1990s a new curriculum, broadly termed 'Gender Studies', was being developed in many universities and colleges in the West. Different versions of gender discourses, centred on emancipatory narratives, sought to deconstruct the complexities of second-wave feminism providing women with ways of envisioning their escape from the dichotomous conceptual gender order that was regarded as the source of women's oppression. Whilst many dedicated gender/ women's studies programmes have now disappeared from the academy, the relevance of gender to understanding the social world has become well established. Avoiding the trap of generalisation about female and male subjectivity has been central to much recent gender research in the fields of sexuality, health, employment as well as in the broader context of political theory and it is this plurality that has helped to maintain the currency of gender as a critical social classification.

The discussion of seminal contributions by early feminist writers to understanding different aspects of gender has been necessarily selective and should be considered alongside other feminist writers mentioned in the previous chapter. This is not a book about feminism per se, but no critique of gender is possible without reference to these early radical feminist ideas that have informed the whole area of gender relations. Much of this early thinking, perhaps understandably, focused on the dichotomous differences between men and women, taking these as a starting point of analysis. Though reference to class, ethnicity and sexuality is made in early feminist literature, the importance of diversity within the social categories women and men is less well-developed and it is to this issue of diversity and heterogeneity that we now turn.

## Diversity

The basis of much early feminist activism is that women have common cause in gender issues such that woman could be understood as a distinct social class particularly in terms of women's *universal* corporeality (Segal, 1999). Indeed, it could be argued that the classification of woman as a class is the most significant contribution of feminism to social theory. Any claims for woman as a homogeneous category, however, soon gave way to understandings of women differentiated by racial, class and ethnic identities as well as by political and sexual loyalties that all help to shape the experience of gender itself. Cott (1986: 58), alluding to the situated beginnings of much second-wave feminist thought, eloquently captures the tensions within the concept 'woman'. She comments "only women holding culturally hegemonic values and positions – that is, in the United States, women who are white, heterosexual, middle class, politically midstream – have the privilege (or deception) of seeing their condition as that of 'woman', glossing over their other characteristics". Race, class, sexuality and gender are inter-related social categories of analysis and connection.

The lived experience of black, working-class women is likely to be culturally and materially different from that of white middle-class women. The lives of lesbian women are different from those of married heterosexual women although, as mothers, women from these differing groups might have more in common with each other than they have with women who do not have children. Similarly, disabled women from different class and racial backgrounds may share more common ground with each other than they can with non-disabled women of any background. These characterisations of difference might, on one level, be seen as simplistic, but they serve to highlight how other socially constructed attributes both heighten and particularise gender identity. The discourse of difference signals the instability of any analysis predicated on an 'all women' approach; it also points to the potential of gender to be a heterogeneous and inclusive conceptual space.

The impacts of class, age, culture and sexual orientation on the experience of gender have been widely reported in a range of writing, both academic and non-academic. Walby (2011), for example, discusses the ways in which feminism impacts on other political projects and is, in turn, changed by them and characterises the resulting adjustments as feminist intersections. She takes a macro perspective focusing on the global issues of nationalism, racism and environmentalism all allied to the wider concern of social justice that aims to deepen democracy and reduce inequality, with the state as a key instrument in achieving these goals. Whilst those issues as global concerns are broader than the scope of this volume, the key precept of intersection as a two-way process is relevant to the current discussion. This is taken up in more depth in Chapter 9 but it is useful here to articulate the mutually constitutive nature of individual and collective subjectivities. Put simply, being a black, lesbian, working-class woman can be seen as an *assemblage* of multiple forms of social inequality. Whether it is useful to empirically separate out any of these features in terms of critically analysing the impact of each is a pragmatic question that, in part, will be dependent on the context. An analysis that can accommodate multiple forms of difference may be ambitious, though Walby (2011: 146) argues that feminist projects successfully use multiple frameworks that they hybridise when this seems more effective.

In some feminist writing the potential for social class to inform the experience of gender has received less attention than race and sexual orientation to the extent that some texts align race (specifically non-whiteness) with class. hooks (2000) seeks to address this conflation in the book *Where we Stand: Class Matters* in which she revisits the construction of social class as a significant independent explanatory factor. hooks argues that classism has undermined feminism through critiques of women's lives on the part of white middle-class women who, with no experience of being marginalised through poverty and/or race, have sought to represent the lives of powerless white and black women. It thus comes as no surprise that some educated black women do not want to make links between their lives and those of white women because of racism (Alibhai-Brown, 2000: 68). hooks (2000) highlights in the US context how women of all races and black men have become the poorest of the poor. Chancer and Watkins (2006) offer a more interwoven discussion of social class through the three paradigms of Marx, Weber and Bourdieu and question the viability of any class paradigm that does not incorporate gender into its analysis. They also caution against simplistic explanatory frameworks specifically to avoid the reduction of both race and gender to a function of class. Instead they argue for the value of multi-dimensionality as a new theoretical tradition to interrogate a range of social complexity in ways similar to those proposed by Walby (2011).

The debate about diversity within feminist analysis relates not only to the key social categories identified above but also has relevance for conceptual strands in feminist thinking. The work of Carol Gilligan (1982) has been particularly significant in demonstrating how feminism has had to embrace multiple approaches to the construction of gender. Her work that argues for recognition and validation of the psychological differences between men and women was seen by some as counter-productive to the efforts and successes of earlier feminism that had called for the elimination of such differences as integral to the equality project. Specifically Gilligan (1982) argued for the valuing of women's nurturing roles that made them more concerned with people than abstractions invoking a feminist morality to shape new approaches to the worlds of politics, science and business – all heavily male-dominated arenas. The underpinning implication of Gilligan's feminist psychological approach is that, given the chance, women do things differently from men – they manage differently, they undertake research from a different standpoint and, crucially, they apply the affective as well as the rational domain to their engagement in the public sphere. At the core of this thesis is the idea that *differently* equals better and more humanely and hers was a challenge to the male way of operating that had come to be viewed as the only way of doing things.

An ethics of care model developed by Gilligan, drawing on principles of connection and subjectivity rather than objective disassociation, sought to reposition the distinct contribution from women. Gilligan's thesis brought centre stage the ethical question of how we treat the other, through focusing on the different values women and men bring to both public problems and intimate relationships. Her ideas that highlight the continuing importance of attachment in the human life cycle (Gilligan, 1982: 23) produced strong and ambivalent reactions from parts of the feminist lobby. Allegations that Gilligan's ideas were helping to reinforce traditional stereotypes of women that historically had been used to limit women's education and employment opportunities were to the fore. Whilst the debate over the claims made by Gilligan still continues, an important consideration is that the claims are not supported by empirical evidence. In the business and management literature, for example, reports of numerous studies aimed at exploring gender differentiated management styles conclude that women and men adopt similar approaches to corporate leadership roles and that, whilst styles may differ, women and men do not use power differently (see, as an example, the work of Carli and Eagly, 2007). Wajcman (1998), who has researched widely on labour market issues, found that the belief that women managers bring a more caring and nurturant style to the job has no currency. Although Gilligan's ideas are contested, they continue to inform ideologies of health and gender and are the subject of further discussion in Chapter 4 that considers men's and women's caring 'careers' that usually begin in the setting of the family.

As discussed in the previous chapter, gender relations are essentially relations of power that operate at a micro level in families as well as at a macro level in institutions such as government, business and religious bodies. Power is discursive and relational and can broadly be defined as the ability of some actors to influence the behaviour of others (Ryle, 2012: 471). Gender categories distribute power in certain ways that generally benefit men over women. Different men, however, may benefit more or less based on their position within other structures of power that ranks some men above others. Whilst as noted above, just as the category woman is diverse and cannot be understood as a homogeneous category, neither is the category man undifferentiated. The question of whether social power is inevitably linked to and invested in 'maleness' has been central to the controversial presumed crisis of masculinity in the West that focuses on men's gender-specific anxieties resulting in the emergence of Masculinities/Men's Studies as a new field of enquiry within the academy (Segal, 1999). The so-called crisis of masculinity is seen as having a number of characteristics. Increasing male unemployment, the lower academic attainment at school of boys than girls, male lower life expectancy and the high rate of suicide among young men are issues that have been identified as contributing to the contemporary malaise of men, (Evans, 2003). Some of these issues, such as lower rates of male life expectancy, have been true for a long time. It is against this background that we have seen a growing interest in men as a separate gendered category.

## Masculinities

Pilcher and Whelan (2004: 82) define masculinity as "the set of social practices and cultural representations associated with being a man". Masculinity can thus be understood as a social system and an identity, both shaped by gendered meanings of manhood strongly associated with men holding some form of social and familial power. Men as fighters and winners, as protectors and providers and as masters and in control are some of the dominant features of 'masculine' manhood. This is a generalisation, but making a clear connection between masculinity and power provides a good starting point for exploration of the diverse and increasingly complex construct that is masculinity. Indeed the subheading above indicates that masculinity takes many forms and the social construction of gender provides a theoretical backdrop for notions of multiple masculinities. Masculinity is historically, culturally and spatially mediated to produce a range of behaviours and intersections with individual men acting out their own definitions of manhood. Masculinity is discursively as well as culturally produced and Coates (2003), for example, provides insight into the ways that talk and the telling of stories, as the symbolic apparatus of society, perform the work of constructing masculinity.

Ways of being a man vary between societies and between different groupings of men within any one society. This plurality, though long acknowledged in the anthropology literature, has in the West been a relatively recent phenomenon. In earlier times the social rules governing the performance of manhood were immutable, allowing for only very limited negotiation in terms of deviation from stereotypical expectations of what it means to be a man. Although historically choices for men have been culturally constrained, this has always been against a background of men having greater access than women to social and material power. The cultural privileges that attach to a normative position for men have, in the main, gone unnoticed, with attention directed more on the disadvantages that attend femininity than questioning the rewards for masculinity. As Lewis and Simpson (2010: 5) comment, gender only gets noticed when it is a source of harm and gender as advantage escapes from view.

Just as in recent years feminism has developed from its Western middle-class origins into a global movement, there has in some Western nations, begun to become established a growing men's movement encouraging men to question both traditional and current gender arrangements. This questioning, as a form of men's consciousness-raising, involved men considering how comfortable or uncomfortable they were with gender power differentials that generally mark relations between men and women, with men, as a social category, benefiting from the 'patriarchal dividend' (Connell, 1995: 79), discussed in the previous chapter. Pilcher and Whelan (2004) explain that some early anti-sexist men's groups wanted to establish a cultural space where they could explore the privileges of patriarchy as well as their responses to this as a demonstration of solidarity with women. Such solidarity was an attempt by some men to acknowledge how they are deeply implicated in existing power structures. Holmes (2009) comments, however, that this solidarity was criticised by some as being merely an exercise in men wanting to feel better about themselves in a personalised way, rather than a commitment to finding solutions to systemic problems.

Another impetus for the movement was the claim by some men that they, as gendered category, needed liberation from masculinity just as women needed to be freed from patriarchy. The analogy with feminism was met with considerable scepticism by some in the feminist movement who took the view that men's liberation could not and should not command the same emancipatory attention accorded to the structural and material inequality of many women's lives. That aside, the connection of the men's movement to feminism was theoretically and empirically reinforced in the project to discuss and reform gender politics. Pilcher and Whelan (2004) comment that members of both the men's and women's movement benefited from mutual collaboration in their wider efforts to confront the oppressive forces of racism and homophobia. Faludi (1991) contests this collaborative emphasis with her theorisation of the men's movement that she argues has its roots, not in a shared project with feminism, but in the defence of hegemonic masculinity as response to the gains made by women and demands from women for men to change. She documents how the men's movement developed into different groupings that included in the US context, the establishment of 'brotherhood lodges' specifically to foster the remasculinising of men who were feeling threatened by the female challenge.

Whilst power differentials mark relations between men and women, they also mark relations among men signalling the importance of avoiding essentialising the category of man (as similarly applies to woman) into a single homogeneous group. Ethnic affiliation, age, class, language, sexual orientation, religion and marital status all rupture the seemingly unified male category. Although male gender identity is created and recreated across the life-course by changing circumstances, most theorising of masculinities has drawn on the experience of younger and middle-aged men, with much attention paid to their embodied selves (Jackson, 2014). However, despite this dominant focus, there is now a developing literature about ageing masculinities as an example of a life-course approach to understanding shifting masculine identities. Focusing on changing masculinities amongst older men, Jackson (2014) comments that loss of social power, bodily strength and reduced status encountered in old age can weaken some ageing men's attachment to patriarchal relations, opening up emancipatory possibilities beyond concerns with work success and competitive individualism. Marginalised by ageism and bodily fragility, many ageing men in Western culture inhabit an ambiguous and contradictory social category (Spector-Mersel, 2006), with this creating barriers to recognising older men as active and complex masculine subjects. This leads Whitehead (2002) to argue that the contradictory mix of privilege, pain, power and fragility to be found in ageing men's lives has not been adequately acknowledged. Reducing what it means to be a man to gender alone, denies the multitude of cross-cultural practices and ideologies that contribute to 'maleness'.

The different ways of 'being a man' are subject to revision and negotiation in contemporary Western society that is gradually moving away from a tendency to see gender demarcations as fixed and purely biologically-based. Though not explored in this volume, the development of new health technologies that make possible gender reassignment, contributes to the diversity and fluidity of gender representations. Masculinity politics are diverse and have come to be interrogated through the sociological concepts of race, class and sexuality in ways similar to the directions taken in feminist theory. Theorisation of masculinity began to take hold in the late 1980s and the work of Segal (1990) that explored the 'masculine ideal' advanced wider thinking about how manliness is constructed, promoted and lived out by individual men and groupings of men. Reflecting on the roles men have as employed workers and fathers and the way that life-course transitions can challenge the performance of manliness, Segal (1990) argued for a theoretical perspective of competing masculinities that she saw as useful in unravelling the 'riddles' of masculinity. Her analysis, for example, of men's use of sexual violence and pornography problematised particular aspects of maleness and was instrumental in extending the debate about the category masculinity that for so long had seemed inherently obscure.

Whilst Segal (1990) had opened up the whole question of manhood as contested and dynamic, it was Bob Connell (1995), in his classic work *Masculinities*, who provided what has come to be regarded as the seminal text on the topic. Space does not allow for a detailed discussion of all of Connell's ideas, but the important concept of hegemonic masculinity developed by Connell merits in-depth scrutiny. The concept and practice of hegemonic masculinity evolved out of a growing recognition of the interplay between gender, race and class giving rise to acknowledgement of multiple masculinities: homosexual as well as heterosexual, black as well as white alongside class-defined masculinities. We should not fall into the trap of oversimplification in respect of these different types of masculinity but these groupings operate on a spectrum of marginalised/privileged masculinity. The co-existence of a range of masculinities thus includes subordinated masculinity experienced by men who challenge the dominant form such as gay men. Another example is that associated with some working-class men – a grotesque masculinity characterised by violence, drinking and out of control and over-weight bodies as articulated by Morgan (1993).

Emerging from this analysis is a particular type of privileged masculinity that is the standard against which all men are judged, even though only a minority of men actually conform to its ideals. This privileged or hegemonic masculinity is largely white, middle class, young and heterosexual; other features include physical fitness and some measure of cultural capital. Holmes (2009: 89) develops this analysis arguing that adhering to this hegemonic form of masculinity "involves having a physically powerful and well-controlled body, a stoic and non-emotional approach to life and, related to that, pursuing power and success in an organised and even ruthless manner". The strictures associated with Connell's model have been explored by a number of commentators leading to some conceptual variations. Sheff (2006), as one example, expands Connell's concept through her examination of men's sexual and romantic interactions in polyamorous relationships. She concludes that hegemonic codes of masculinity are subject to reconfiguration and adaptation such that hegemonic masculinity is lived out in diverse ways and is thus not a wholly unified concept or practice. It is nuanced and contextualised. However, though diverse male hegemonic codes have emerged, the principle of compulsory heterosexuality remains pre-eminent.

Rejection of all things feminine and the homosexual, both being in opposition to real manliness, is central to accomplishing displays of hegemonic masculinity. Because the primary audience for this heightened performance of masculinity is other men, it is imperative that there is no hint of emotional attachment to men as this could be perceived as sexual interest in men that goes beyond the acceptable display of camaraderie or collegiality often present within sport and workplaces. In this model, being homosexual makes the achievement of real manhood impossible.

Because of class-based as well as race-based experiences of relative powerlessness evoking feelings of alienation, some men take out their frustration and resentment about their devalued social position on women, sometimes in extremely violent ways. This violence, often in the domestic sphere, enables men to regain a sense of control in their lives because they have relative power over their wives/partners who may be economically dependent and/or caring for children. Male powerlessness in the public sphere is compensated for by reinforcing power in the private sphere. This form of marginalised masculinity could be understood as a strategy used by some men to avoid emasculation. It is important to note that while other issues such as drug or alcohol use may be additional explanatory factors for men's damaging behaviour, marginalised masculinity amongst some men, involving low self-esteem, is now recognised in the social policy literature to be of pivotal importance. Ryle (2012) contends that men are engaged in an ongoing project of defending themselves against emasculation; if that is the case it is not difficult to see how violence can be a marker of some forms of masculinity. The pressure to reinforce masculine identity involves a constant self-scrutiny, again particularly in presentation of self to other men. This impression management is always context specific and subject to other features of social stratification.

Consideration of the part played by race in confirming a particular type of male identity is discussed by Alexander (2002) in her ethnography of young black masculinity in the British context. The importance of the peer group as a collective identity that, in the face of frustration, failure and racial rejection, operates as a primary source of socialisation for black youth is drawn out to document the emergence of a particular form of male subculture in response to wider social rejection. Alexander (2002: 92) notes that: "subcultural groups are usually regarded as internally homogeneous and positioned in direct opposition to an overarching hegemonic order which constitutes 'society'". The development of 'black macho' emerges as a distinct form of young masculinity directed at reinforcing group norms as resistance to perceived dominant external structures of oppression. Attributes of this masculinity relate to performative aspects in terms of dress style, dance prowess, the ability to 'talk your own story' and, most crucially, the ability to assert physical control should the need arise. All of these performances were directed towards attracting women, with competitiveness inflecting the internal dynamics of the group. Heteronormativity was found similarly to be central to young black masculine identity in a US study of poor black teenage men conducted by Froyum (2007). Dissociation from gay-coded behaviour and strict conformity to heterosexist ideologies by black men in the study eliminated the risk of them being perceived as anything other than confirmed heterosexual males, with being gay seen as being at the bottom of the social hierarchy.

Internal relations within the group studied in Alexander's (2002) project, though not always harmonious, were regulated primarily in terms of pressure from external forces seen as potentially emasculating. Images of young black masculinity discussed in this study call attention to one display of black male identity and do not constitute wider representativeness. Segal (1990) comments that, whilst oppositional meaning has been inherent in shaping understandings and experiences of black masculinity, being a black male has increasingly become characterised by diversity rather than 'sameness'. Obama's election in 2008 to the role of US President, as a black man, helped fuel the debate about opportunity and fulfilment of individual potential across the race/class divide. Much of the associated rhetoric, however, has remained at the level of theory and ideology rather than advancing policy-making and culture change, with Obama's presidency coinciding with black America's economic descent (*Guardian*, 3 November 2012).

Oppositional meaning, identified by Segal (1990) as being integral to male black identity, has also influenced the social construction of gay masculinity that has been the subject of extensive theorising in the academy. Evans (2003: 59), commenting on the continuing cultural dominance of heterosexuality in discursive masculinity, notes that "homosexuality [has] maintained its status as a practice defined by its difference from heterosexuality rather than being distinct in itself". Whether or not this claim would find widespread support amongst social commentators in the current climate of neoliberal sexual politics, it does usefully point to the way in which homosexuality defined as 'other', has normative heterosexuality as the benchmark against which it is judged. Hocquengham (1972) reinforces opposionality as integral to homosexuality suggesting that this form of sexuality is the opposite of identity, being desire and practice that cannot be blended into a unified sense of self. This is a complex area and insights from the fields of psychology and anthropology contribute wider understanding to the nature of both heterosexuality and homosexuality as perverse and fluctuating and subject to contradiction.

As noted above, the concept of hegemonic masculinity developed by Connell (1995) has been a powerful influence in constructing a mainstream privileged type of masculinity. It has also been instrumental in positioning gay liberation as an explicit alternative to heterosexual masculinity, particularly the hegemonic form. Gay identities are diverse and have been theorised in terms of particular features such as recognition of male tenderness (culturally a feminine attribute), adoption of hyper-masculine lifestyles (body building is one feature) and political activism in support of gay equality. Alongside, some forms of gay masculinity have come to be associated with particular sexual practices such as sadomasochism that Chaline (2010) argues has a long established place in gay culture. Whilst some popular notions of gay identity position this form of masculinity as classless, Heaphy (2011) argues for an analysis that incorporates socio-economic factors to counter the idea of gay class transcendence. Although traditional concepts of family are deemed to exclude gay (lesbian and homosexual) parenting, gay fatherhood is another form of masculinity that has gradually gained social currency and this, despite long running discourses associating gay parenting with "dangerous queerness" (Smith, 1992). Stacey (2006) documents narratives of gay parental desire that elucidate the challenges to gay paternity and the successful reconfiguring of gay parenthood in creative ways. However, writing in the context of Spain that in recent times has experienced significant social and legal change, Pichardo (2011) uncovers different forms of discrimination and homophobic prejudice connected to the legitimising of same-sex headed families. Fathering, whether gay or heterosexual, involves competing definitions of masculinity and is a subject we will return to in later chapters.

## Conclusion

The discussion in this chapter has focused on the ways in which sociological theory, drawing mainly on feminist ideas, has critically examined the sex/gender identity, moving this beyond fixed or 'natural' categories. Insights from anthropology and psychology have also featured in the discussion to strengthen perspectives of the diversity of the sex/gender system that, in Western societies, is still understood mainly in terms of mutually exclusive hierarchical categories characterised by a system of patriarchal structures. Eschewing ephemerality, feminism has been able to claim many achievements in advancing gender equality and this has given rise to what can best be termed as 'backlash' critiques (see Faludi, 1991). These return gender to a close association with the biological to suggest that feminist thinking, straining against the inevitable forces of the 'natural', holds only limited validity and, therefore, should be discredited. Backlash agendas have emerged precisely because the conceptualisation of gender has been so successful, particularly in its theorisation of patriarchy.

Patriarchy has not disappeared and the relevance of gender has material significance beyond the level of theory. The critical application of gender theory to understanding our daily lives, our rights as women and men and access to opportunities to develop and fulfil our potential, is relevant across all spheres. Whilst I argue for an overarching gender perspective to explain experiences of health and working in healthcare roles, it is not my intention to underplay the genuine dilemmas and tensions between gender equality and cultural autonomy. Nor do I set out to mask how race and class impact on women's and men's lives and the above critique of diversity within gendered categories serves to demonstrate how power is mediated through a range of social differences. Indeed, it has become increasingly clear that the assertion of oppositional categories of difference such as black/white, for example, tends to create fixed positions that result in another version of the suppression of difference. Internal coherence within categories is not only theoretically unsustainable, it is materially deceptive. Current feminist activism is increasingly attuned to the impact of a range of intersecting differences that can underlie oppression. Making activist and political space to draw attention to the ways in which marginalisation is created and experienced in terms of class, race, age, ability, sexuality as well as gender, has become central to the feminist project. These concerns are considered further in Chapter 9, which has intersectionality as its theme.

In the next chapter ideas about the socially constructed nature of gender categories are elaborated in relation to women and men's experience of health and illness. This is a burgeoning area of study that within the discipline of medical sociology encompasses theoretical, policy and empirical directions, all of which contribute to an ongoing debate about the classic problems associated with health politics characterised by issues of personal choice and distribution of scarce resources.

# Chapter 3
# Women's and Men's Health

## Introduction

Across the many dimensions of health that include mental health reproductive/sexual health and death and dying, much has been written about the ways in which gender affects health and illness. Gender and its impact on women's and men's experience of health and illness is a huge topic. Biological differences between the sexes are important but aspects of gender relations that are also significant relate to resources, health behaviour and healthcare. Features of diversity such as class, ethnicity and sexuality all help to further explain the health status and health experiences of women and men. Whilst the gendering of healthcare roles is considered in Chapters 4 and 5, the focus in the current chapter is on how women and men view and experience health. Although the emphasis of the discussion that follows is on gender differences, Robertson (2007: 23) usefully reminds us that research into health and gender is increasingly showing more similarities than differences in physical morbidity amongst women and men, certainly up until the age of 70. Despite this growing convergence, a number of significant gender health differences remains, with for example, Pietila and Rytkonen (2008: 1070) commenting that "health is not a man's domain".

Women live longer than men and are more likely to use healthcare services and engage in help-seeking behaviour (such as screening) in relation to health concerns. They are also more likely to be both the paid and unpaid carers of the chronically ill and dying (Field et al., 1997; Segal, 2013). Men engage more heavily in risky behaviours such as smoking and drinking and are more likely to have unhealthy diets and take less exercise and be candidates for heart surgery (Payne, 2006). Men of working age receive greater attention from hospital staff and are more likely than women to be informed of their terminal diagnosis (Field et al., 1997). Mental health problems are far more prevalent among women who are more likely than men to self-harm in ways that are not fatal (Featherstone et al., 2007: 133). Men, on the other hand, are more likely to die through suicide (Busfield, 2010; Johnson et al., 2012; Warwick-Booth et al., 2012) with the related point argued by Jaworski (2014: 3) that 'gender is central to understanding suicide'. Mental distress is much less understood in men than in women (Ridge et al., 2011) and Ryle (2012: 298) comments that, because depression is seen predominantly as a feminine disease by both sufferers and clinicians, men are far less likely to seek medical help for their depression. The paid employment that women and men undertake is another determinant of health, with more men than women experiencing long-term health problems due to both accidents at work and the physically hazardous nature of some working environments. The masculinised male gender role, imbued with a sense that men should not 'give in' to illness, culturally restricts men's use of health services (Noone and Stephens, 2008).

These opening summary headline comments provide a snapshot of some of the key differences in women's and men's health behaviours that Saltonstall (1993) argues are shaped by social norms influencing individual behaviour seen as appropriately male or female. In that sense, Saltonstall (1993: 12) contends, "the doing of health is a form of doing gender". Charmaz (1995) supports this position with her claim that a gender identity can be strengthened or diminished through experiencing illness. Help-seeking and a more protected status are part of conventional ideas about female roles. Men, on the other hand, are expected to deny illness, be more self-reliant and avoid asking for help – this characterisation is termed by Riska (2002: 34) as 'hardy man' and by del Mar Garcia-Calvente et al. (2012) as 'tough man'. Gender beliefs contribute to men's healthcare avoidance and Charteris-Black and Seale (2010), exploring how gender influences the language of illness in terms of male and female illness narratives, found that men's accounts of serious illness tend towards avoidance, abstraction and emotional distancing whereas those of women are more emotionally direct and often represent illness as personally transformative. This reinforces the popular discourse of the 'male deficit' model whereby men cannot easily express their feelings or verbalise their experience of illness. It also positions women as better able than men to manage illness with this aligned to the norms of femininity. However, Charteris-Black and Seale (2010) stress the importance of not over-generalising, particularly as their empirical research uncovered significant variation within gender groups. For example, higher-status and younger men are more likely to adopt the more emotional vocabulary associated with 'modern' masculinity.

The implication that men are emotionally disconnected from their bodies as evidenced by these behaviours is now starting to be challenged. For example, Robertson et al. (2010) question men's perceived wholly functional mechanistic and sometimes dismissive view of their bodies. A more complex dynamic involving men in risk-taking and macho stoicism on the one hand and active health-seeking on the other is contributing to the notion of masculinities in transition, as argued for by Robinson and Hockey (2011). Although clearly important, a solely gender-based explanation of health in isolation from other social variables is empirically inadequate. Whilst women, as a category, live longer than men, males from the upper social classes will live longer than women from lower socio-economic groups. They will also experience less ill-health over the life-course. Inequalities in health are also a matter of geography and Graham's (2009) analysis describes how neighbourhoods appear to influence health, over and above the social characteristics of the local population. Macintyre et al. (2002) develop this point arguing that place, as a determinant of health, has been under-theorised and should be more strongly incorporated within analyses of individual and community health that inform policy and practice.

The ways in which women and men experience health that includes responses to illness, are now explored through a series of case studies drawn from the disciplines of medical sociology and anthropology. The material presented highlights how health, rather than a gender-neutral construct, is very much shaped by gender difference as well as by wider cultural health discourses. Health and healthcare were and continue to be major concerns of second-wave feminists giving rise to the practice of women's health politics that has become increasingly global in its focus reflecting the more general growth of international collaboration in women's politics (Doyal, 1996). Insights from feminist theory have much to offer in extending understanding of the mechanics of gender that go beyond theoretical conceptualisations to both inform and explain the health careers of women and men. The oppressive role of patriarchy in shaping the lives of women, discussed in the previous two chapters, provides a useful theoretical canvas against which to explore the issue of women's reproductive health. This has been characterised largely by professional relationships between female patients and male clinicians that disempower women within established hierarchies of social control. Other case studies in the chapter will report the experience of breast cancer in women, gendered aspects of HIV/AIDS and men's cancer health concerns that increasingly are the subject of scrutiny within masculinities studies.

## Women and reproduction

Women's reproductive rights have been and continue to be an important focus of activism within the women's health movement that has campaigned to bring women the right to control their fertility. The right to contraception, safe abortion, non-medicalised birth and access to fertility treatment are issues that have been widely discussed in the feminist and medical sociology literature. Much of this discussion has centred on the politics of choice, specifically increasing choice for women through which they can gain [some] control over their biology. This, however, is a contested domain with often competing interests captured by Pascall (1997: 166) who explains that "regulating reproduction is a matter of the most private choice and the most public interest". The use of a range of reproductive technologies is seen to have contributed to enhancing choice for women and has become an established feature of modern medicine. In particular, infertility has come to be regarded as a growing health problem and assisted reproductive technologies such as IVF, whilst medicalising the experience of involuntary childlessness for many couples, have also increased the potential of parenthood for some (Heitman, 2002).

These technological advances, however, have not been universally welcomed and this is very much a contested area within feminist writing. Analysing reproductive technologies within broader social power relations, some commentators interpret these technologies as liberating for women whilst others argue that they serve the interests of patriarchal science and medicine resulting in women's loss of agency and knowledge. As an example, in the context of male-dominated science and medicine, techniques such as IVF can represent an increase in men's control over women's bodies (Pilcher and Whelan, 2004). These ideas are part of the wider debate about gender, technology and health that is the subject of Chapter 6. For the current chapter's discussion, it is useful to highlight that technology is an important cultural component of reproduction that is constructed as a social institution with systems of governance and regulatory regimes centred on 'producing' and 'managing' pregnant bodies (Ettorre and Kingdom, 2010).

The relationship between the female body and procreation is an enduring feature of dominant discourses of womanhood. The possibility of disrupting the procreation story through the availability of medically supervised legal abortion has led to the emergence of a new cultural script for women who, in most countries of the West, now have access to safe abortion. Abortion, along with contraception, has fostered a critical realignment of women's reproductive health that challenges the cultural dominance of reproduction and motherhood in the female life-course. The tendency to see reproduction as a site of oppression and motherhood as a burden, from which women should be liberated, was a feature of early second-wave feminist thought (Rich, 1976). Only later were the positive attributes of motherhood articulated by feminist commentators.

What was crucial was the possibility that women could have reproductive choice even if they had little influence over the conditions of childbirth and the social control of motherhood. Although reproductive choice for women is now widely accepted as a right, its adoption within healthcare systems has not been universal and is still subject to cultural and legal restriction in many countries, including some in the West (Ryle, 2012).

Nowhere is the politics of abortion more polarised than in the United States that has seen the divergent positions of the pro-life and pro-choice movements become a deeply entrenched battleground of a rights-based discourse. Ginsburg (2006), in her ethnography about the establishment in the American state of North Dakota of a Woman's Health centre to publically offer abortions, highlights how competing 'life' discourses are invoked to define women on either side of the argument. This is rich ideological polemical territory. Broadly sketched, women supporting the pro-life movement perceived abortion to be a secular intrusion to undermine family life and reshape women into structural men. The privileging of sexual pleasure and individual ambition disconnected from procreation, renders women as culturally male and destroys nurturance that is the essence of womanliness. Pro-choice supporters in Ginsburg's (2006) study saw access to choice as an expression of women's freedom and ability to determine this aspect of their life and also as a way of overcoming sexual discrimination. Ginsburg (2006) contends that at the nexus of the debate over reproductive choice, is the ambivalence of motherhood, with pro-life arguments pointing to the achievement of nurturance in motherhood *despite* ambivalent feelings. This is contrasted with the pro-choice position that is seen to stress the other side of ambivalence with abortion providing a framework for organising *disorderly* life transitions. These dichotomous positions on abortion have been rehearsed in other contexts beyond the US and serve to illustrate opposed, but inter-related, paradigms of ways of being female.

A further aspect of women's experience of reproductive health that has come under the critical gaze of medical sociologists in recent years is that of childbirth. The conceptualisation of childbirth as a regulatory regime has its roots in feminist scholarship that has identified ways in which the pregnant body is subject to surveillance and control by the medical profession. Whilst the value of medicine within maternity care is acknowledged (in, for example, monitoring foetal health risks), the emphasis on medical management of pregnancy that in turn is viewed as intrinsically pathological and, therefore, risky has been increasingly questioned by feminist scholars. Ettorre and Kingdom (2010), for example, identify the increase in caesarean deliveries that, they argue, reflects obstetric attitudes rather than clinical need. Planned caesarean section rather than a vaginal delivery, as an elective choice, has become available in many countries.

Some might argue that elective caesarean delivery, as a planned medical procedure, is one way of women reclaiming control of the birth process with convenience and predictability of the temporal dimension providing differential practical benefits to themselves, their partners and their employers. Other physiological benefits are maintenance of the pelvic floor and the aesthetic advantage of less pronounced 'stretch marks', both promoting gendered feminine ideals. Whilst caesarean section may remove some of the uncertainties of vaginal childbirth, especially for older first-time mothers, an implication of its increased use is the potential for this procedure to be adopted as a norm, particularly with the rise in litigation throughout healthcare. Turner (2004) thus notes that with pressure on maternity services, obstetricians are more likely to opt for caesarean delivery whenever a complication arises. This has resource implications and also carries the potential to devalue the skills and knowledge of midwives, the majority of whom are women.

It is important to be aware that pregnant bodies and childbirth are gendered sites and subject to cultural processes both within and outside medicine (Oakley, 1984). The gendered management of childbirth has a long and mixed history that Donnison (1988) traces from the Middle Ages through to the twentieth century. She notes that whilst women midwives acted as birth attendants in the sixteenth and seventeenth centuries in Europe, the eighteenth century saw their decline in this role and gradual replacement by male midwives more in the role of medical men. It was not until the twentieth century and the certification of midwifery practice, that we see women again taking up this occupation that was regarded as an appropriate way for unsupported gentlewomen to earn a livelihood. Increasingly midwifery has come to be seen as a distinctly female occupation, but one heavily imbued with medical values, particularly in hospital consultant units (Donnison, 1988). Donnison (1988: 203) thus argues that although midwives are the senior person present in three quarters of all deliveries, "*she* has declined to little more than a handmaiden of the obstetrician and a minder of *his* machines". Wajcman (1991) supports this claim specifically drawing out the contested relations between midwives, technology and obstetricians.

Discussion of control of the pregnant body and the birth process has long been a concern of feminists with Oakley (1984: 11) arguing that the care of pregnant women has been and remains contested expert territory. The main contribution of feminist theory in this area has been recognition of the powerful interplay between culture, modern medicine and women's bodies. Rich (1976), writing in the early period of second-wave feminism, saw the male cultural rules surrounding pregnancy and mothering as alienating of women and as counter to the experience of motherhood that can be both pleasurable and empowering for women. Pregnancy and childbirth are not gender-neutral processes and discourses of stylish, fashionable and active 'fit' pregnancy, endorsing an idealised normative pregnant form, are now to be found as part of popular media narratives. Advice to pregnant women about what they should eat and drink and how they should exercise has come (mainly) from male doctors (Freedman, 2001), contributing to the male controlled social institution of motherhood. Such discourses are simplistic and deny the diversity of pregnancy that includes the experience of disabled pregnant women and those women whose cultural backgrounds require them to perform pregnancy out of the public gaze as much as possible – because it is through the body that social concerns are often symbolically enacted (Eilberg-Schwartz, 1990: 117). An example of how cultural beliefs may impact on the experience and outcome of pregnancy is highlighted by Sheaff (2005: 213) in relation to British Pakistani women. He notes that there is low utilisation of prenatal screening amongst this group largely because of unawareness amongst this community that medical procedures such as screening are not subject to religious prohibition.

## Breast cancer – a female disease of the modern age

Cancer is a complex group of diseases that have been present in ancient as well as modern societies though, because cancer is predominantly a disease of older age, cancer is more prominent in modern populations that, in the West, are characterised by increased longevity. The causes of cancer are as varied as the cancers themselves with some, such as lung cancer, associated with particular risk factors such as smoking. Although discussion of the epidemiology of cancer is beyond the scope of this volume, it is relevant to note that because of better recording systems, we now have a more developed understanding of the incidence of cancer as a global health problem. Each year WHO (World Health Organisation) publishes figures of cancer deaths worldwide as well as trends in disease type and its figures show that breast cancer ranks first or second in female cancer incidence in every major region of the world (WHO, 2013).

The prime aim of the discussion that follows is to reveal the meanings that breast cancer has in contemporary society as a way of exposing the deeply gendered dimensions of the disease. Though not exclusively a women's health issue (some men are diagnosed with breast cancer), the disease now has a well-developed ideological and discursive terrain characterised by the many stories of breast cancer told by women with the condition. Perhaps more than any other disease, the experience of breast cancer has been recounted through film, television, (auto)biography, fiction and the daily press in what is now a vast amount of personal and social commentary. Activism around breast cancer is also a source of published accounts of the ways in which the disease affects not only those who have it, but their families and social networks. With increased research into treatment of breast cancer and better long-term survival rates, the dominant ideology of breast cancer has, in recent years, moved towards a paradigm of progress, improvement and choice in respect of treatment options (Potts, 2000; Twomey, 2012). As part of the improvement narrative, emphasis on genetic factors, more individually targeted treatment, diet and reconstruction has helped shape a thriving cancer industry and this, not just in relation to breast cancer, but other cancers too. Pharmaceutical and biotechnology companies, research organisations, dedicated cancer charities and clinicians contribute to the high-volume and financially lucrative business of cancer.

The widespread implementation of mass breast screening programmes in the name of health promotion has persuaded many women of the need for regular surveillance of their breasts. These screening programmes, developed mainly by men, are seen by some feminist commentators such as Simpson (2000) as a form of compliance for women. However, mammograms, as the screening procedure is termed, are generally effective in identifying early stage breast cancer (Friedman et al., 2012). Despite this, the procedure has come under considerable negative scrutiny in relation to increasing women's level of anxiety, particularly where they are recalled for further examination when abnormalities or lumps are detected. Blow et al. (2011) highlight the intensely emotional nature of the time before recall. Knowledge about benign breast disease and its risk significance relative to the development of malignant breast disease has thrown up a number of uncertainties, mainly due to the lack of standardised criteria for classifying benign conditions (Gifford, 2002). Gifford (2002) notes that for women risk is experienced as a condition of non-health, placing them at risk of further medicalisation that Kearney (2006) argues is also perceived as a threat to their femininity. Within contemporary medicine one cannot be both healthy and at risk at the same time. This is discussed in more detail in Chapter 7 that focuses on the topic of health promotion.

The experience of having breast cancer has been the subject of a number of personal accounts from women in high profile positions as well as from women out of the public eye. The accounts vary in their structure, intensity and language but a common theme is the sensitivity expressed in relation to the bodily site of the disease – the female breast. Inevitably the disease is seen as a women's health issue; it is also a sexualised illness with the breast a site of sexual pleasure. Allied to this are the dominant discourses of femininity and maternal role associated with the breast. Multiple representations attach to the breast as iconic; the erotic potential of the fetishised breast is contrasted with the nurturing, life-giving maternal breast. These meanings illustrate how the breast is contested embodiment and how breast cancer is framed by cultural understandings and gendered conceptions of idealised womanhood. Breast cancer is especially culturally-laden because of the way in which femininity is located in the female body that historically has been sexualised for the male gaze and masculine consumption. Feminist thinking has critically analysed how the female body, as commodified object, is the currency by which women are socially valued. However, the cancerous breast is neither sexy nor maternal and the potential for either of these attributes is culturally eliminated through the onset of the disease. It comes, then, as no surprise that stories of women with breast cancer having radical surgery in the form of a mastectomy situate their post-operative identity in terms of a mutilated femininity (Saywell et al., 2000).

Some of these issues are drawn out in the story told by Dina Rabinovitch (2007) who, at the age of 42, was diagnosed with breast cancer at a time when she was still breast-feeding her youngest child. An orthodox Jew living in London and married for the second time following a bitter divorce, Rabinovitch recounts the emotional and practical struggle of being a 'younger' breast cancer sufferer, with a large re-formed family to care for as well as a career as a journalist to continue. The importance to her of fashion, looking good and maintaining her femininity is threaded through her cancer story. "They call this the fashionable cancer", she wrote after her mastectomy, "but nobody's tackling the basic fashion question: what do you wear?". As she prepares for a magazine piece about post-mastectomy clothes, Rabinovitch is aided by a young male stylist who asks her why she declines to wear a prosthesis. She responds that it feels humiliating, uncomfortable and fake. Only an authentic female body will do. Authenticity is synonymous with the 'normal' sexualised female form. Commenting on the dilemma of choosing suitable clothes during the hot summer of 2006, a year before she was to die, Rabinovitch (2007) writes: "This hot summer *Gap* comes to the rescue, producing sorbet-coloured lines of sleeveless, thin cotton, that I buy in reams and wear sliced one over the other, the thinness making the heat bearable, the different colours and the layers letting me not look like a freak".

The conjunction between fashion and breast cancer is critiqued by Cartwright (1998) who argues that the aesthetic emphasis through fashion in relation to the disease, signifies a cultural preoccupation with the bodily site of the illness. The procedure of breast reconstruction contributes to this aesthetic dimension of breast cancer that is experienced physiologically and emotionally in different ways by the women afflicted. Whilst breasts are not central to every woman's sense of female gender identity, for many women a radically altered appearance resulting from the removal of one or both breasts may be difficult to come to terms with. Surgical removal of the breasts is seen as radical because it is unavoidably public. Whilst breast reconstruction can help to restore 'normal' appearance and self-confidence, a woman's 'new' body may not feel natural and the reconstruction can cause restriction in movement giving rise to discomfort and physical awkwardness (Hallowell, 2000). Some women's accounts in Hallowell's (2000) study report an improved sense of self through reconstruction because of their better-shaped and 'younger' *new* breasts contributing to an enhanced rather than compromised feminine identity, particularly in relation to sexual attractiveness.

Ruth Picardie (1998) describes breast cancer from a different perspective. Hers is a less breast-centred self-reflective account infused with humour, resentment and bitter irony focusing on the unglamorous raw nature of the illness and strategies of resistance – she remarks "at least stroppy cows live longer" (Picardie, 1998: 31). In her breast cancer story the mythology of cancer heroism is elided. Instead, she viscerally recounts how hair loss, weight gain, burn marks from radiotherapy, vomiting and endless waiting for the 'big day', as a terminally ill person, all position her at the crossroads between life and death. In her case, expectations of dramatic weight loss to make her fade away were countered by weight gain that made her look well (fat) in a post-chemotherapy body that defied notions of gendered slim feminine beauty. Focus on the breast obscures other dimensions of the gendered breast cancer experience and culturally polices how women with the disease *should* experience their bodies. The assumption that mastectomies must be hidden and that breast reconstruction is mandatory to avoid "failed beauty" (Boulton and Malacrida, 2012: 511), illustrates the heavily gendered representation of the disease.

The breast as danger and affirmation in terms of female gender identity is an underpinning epistemological theme in the breast cancer narrative. Breast cancer is visually and culturally coded to signify female embodiment as a site of contested meanings. Breast cancer, though both shared and unique experience, is situated amidst patterns and trends of disease presentation that has given rise to a well-developed prevention and treatment narrative considered in more detail in Chapter 7.

## HIV/AIDS

Just when we thought antibiotics, the contraceptive pill and more liberal attitudes had taken the danger and chagrin out of sexual behaviour, the arrival out of nowhere in the early 1980s of HIV/AIDS – an incurable, fatal and highly contagious sexual disease, challenged medical science and triggered a public health crisis, particularly in the US. Because of the association of AIDS with the sexual behaviour of gay men, the emerging AIDS 'epidemic' amongst this population gave rise to an ensuing moral panic. The concept of a "sick society" (Lock, 2002: 195), with an allied threat to the prevailing moral order, was widely invoked in public narratives. The disease, culturally defined and mediated through discourses of risk, came to be characterised by the 'polluting' sexual practices of gay men resulting in their stigmatisation. "Naming a risk amounts to an accusation" (Douglas, 2002: xix) and the resulting negative labelling of HIV as the 'gay plague' and the 'gay cancer' (Warwick-Booth et al., 2012: 121), have continued the cultural link between the disease and gay men.

HIV and AIDS within media narratives are very much associated with lifestyle choice, particularly gay lifestyles and explanations of causation are heavily value-laden. Behavioural traits of self-indulgence, lack of self-discipline, high-risk sexual practices and out of control sexual desire contribute to the ideology of the disease as social deviance. The incidence of the disease amongst sex workers and injecting drug users, also seen as moral transgressors of socially accepted behavioural norms, has further heightened the cultural stigmatisation for those diagnosed as HIV positive making them vulnerable to discrimination. The notion that AIDS somehow punishes socially marginalised people is a feature of some social commentary on the disease. Individuals who contract the virus after receiving infected blood generally escape blame, as theirs is not perceived as illness-causing behaviour.

AIDS is now a leading cause of death among men and women across the world and, whilst culturally and empirically linked to unsafe sex practices, it has come to be increasingly theorised not only as a medical issue but as one shaped by social inequality and, in the global context, by the politics of development. Although AIDS is now recognised as a disease affecting a wide population and not just gay men, within the gay community, AIDS has had a profound impact on perceptions of health. Robertson (2007) argues that amongst gay men, health is increasingly understood and defined through the lens of sexual health, specifically being AIDS-free. Although prior to the AIDS pandemic in the 1980s, an embryonic gay men's health movement existed, it was the emergence of AIDS that gave it momentum and focus. Drawing inspiration from feminism, an analysis linking the social position of gay men (specifically their gendered existence) and their health began to emerge. However, Edwards (2010) argues that because the focus of the gay men's health movement has been on HIV/AIDS, this has highlighted sexuality and obscured gender. The construction of gay male health as being synonymous with sexual health has been dominated by the rhetoric of risk at both the individual and 'group' level. Robertson (2007) outlines how the material relationship between gay male health and risk is part of wider gendered discourses around masculinity and risk that he contends are culturally situated along a spectrum of 'machoness'. Some behaviour such as unprotected anal sex between gay men termed as 'barebacking' (Frasca et al., 2012: 946), whilst being high-risk, may enhance a 'macho' identity. This promotion of 'masculinity' over health may, of course, apply equally in the heterosexual context.

In the West AIDS has become a chronic condition that, through the use of anti-retroviral drugs, can be managed on a long-term basis. In a potential post-AIDS world (in terms of certain death from the disease), Baer et al. (2003), drawing on a study conducted in San Francisco, report the view of HIV-negative men who see AIDS as more of an inconvenience than a killer. HIV-positive men in the same study commented that they were no longer warning their friends to take care over AIDS. The resulting increase in unsafe sex practices such as reduced condom use, particularly among young gay men, many of who advocated this as 'better' or more erotic sex, has led to a reported rise in the numbers of gay men diagnosed as HIV-positive and this following a sustained period of declining prevalence (Guy et al., 2007).

The association of HIV and AIDS with gay sexuality and in particular with casual gay sexual encounters endures due, at least in part, to the well-established cultural machinery of homophobic politics. But this is only one aspect of the gendered terrain of the disease. Gilbert and Selikow (2010), focusing on the gendered distribution of the virus from a global perspective, argue that, although the emergence of AIDS was initially associated with gay men, there now is an increasing feminisation of AIDS in the developing world, with its extent varying from region to region. Globally, women account for half of all HIV infections, a percentage that has remained stable in recent years (Gilbert and Selikow, 2010). This level of infection amongst women demonstrates that HIV is not confined to the sub-groups of gay men, intravenous drug users and those involved in transactional sex – it is a generalised heterosexual epidemic.

In many parts of the developing world, women's socio-economic position is determined by their dependency on men rendering women as socially powerless. Gilbert and Selikow (2010) cite the situation in South Africa as a case study through which to explore a number of gendered subject positions in the experience of HIV and AIDS. Exposed to what Gilbert and Selikow (2010: 194) term as "dangerous masculinities" characterised by violence and the insistence of having multiple and concurrent sexual partners, women find themselves unable to negotiate condom use. In this context men may regard condom use as compromising of their virility and sexual pleasure, with women forced to comply even though this may increase their risk of HIV infection. Sex is culturally constructed and the extent to which sexual practices in the context of a male-dominated society are subject to revision, redefinition and negotiation by women, is a function of gendered power relations.

The further impact of HIV/AIDS on women concerns the role they have in caring for orphaned children and other family members who are infected with the virus and this, frequently when they are ill themselves. Because of the prevailing ideology that care is the responsibility of women, many women, young and old, are shouldering a disproportionate burden of care for those dying from AIDS. Some women are undertaking this work as part of a professional nursing role but many are not and, unsupported and unrecognised, are providing community-based care, often with very little input from public health services. For some women, the informal caring role becomes a full-time occupation such that they have to stop their paid work. A move into poverty is the consequence.

The support of those dying from AIDS in South Africa has in recent times become the concern of the palliative care movement, with attendant gender implications. The South Coast Hospice (SCH) located in the province of Kwazulu-Natal in South Africa, provides palliative care to a highly disadvantaged and impoverished population where there is 70 per cent unemployment and where the prevalence of tuberculosis is 116 per 100,000 (Defellippi and Mnguni, 2009). However, it is the scale of HIV/AIDS in the area that has been the key challenge, with the social and psychological trauma associated with the disease for both sufferers and their carers an overwhelming problem. With anti-retroviral medication only very recently becoming available in South Africa, the hospice had to plan services with the prospect of huge numbers of AIDS patients requiring palliative care. Much of their work, therefore, involves the use of lay volunteers to help provide integrated community home care. This high level of lay support has become necessary because the traditional care safety net of the extended family system in South Africa is being eroded by HIV/AIDS (Defellippi and Mnguni, 2009). Overburdened grandmothers, often frail and underfed, cannot cope with caring alone for their own sick adult children and young grandchildren and many have to develop a range of livelihood strategies to support themselves and those for whom they care (Wangui, 2009).

Nearly all the volunteers at SCH are women. In addition, a majority (60 per cent) of AIDS patients referred to the hospice are women who have contracted the virus from a male partner to whom they have been faithful, with the result that the skill level required by volunteers to initiate discussion about sexual health problems with both the infected person and their partner is very high. This is challenging work because, as Auger (2007) opines, HIV/AIDS is first and foremost a sociological issue with issues of stigma and social exclusion never far from view.

## Male cancers

Discussion of cancers that impact specifically on men is part of wider understandings of men's health that now has a separately defined constituency comprising both biological and social factors. Broadly sketched, male reproductive characteristics that are biologically determined and, engagement in the male role or masculine practices that are socially determined, are the two elements that comprise this constituency (Schofield, 2010). The assertion that men have a collective interest and identity in relation to health status is contested because, as highlighted in the previous chapter man, as a social category, is highly differentiated through class, ethnicity and sexuality – all influencing the performance of masculinities. However, male as a biologically sex-differentiated category from woman, serves as a lens through which to explore male-specific disease processes such as those of prostate and testicular cancer. Given the cultural emphasis on the centrality of male genitals to sexuality and essentialised masculinity, there are some important psycho-social implications of these cancers, some of which are discussed below.

Prostate cancer is predominantly a disease of older age mainly affecting men over 50 and one that in recent years has become more prominent in health promotion discourses that in earlier times gave only scant attention to the condition. The prostate is a small gland found only in men, important for sexual and reproductive functioning. It produces a unique protein which is the basis for the commonly termed 'PSA test', a simple blood test that is used to detect malignant prostatic disease (Faulkner, 2012: 222). The attitudes of men to being tested for prostate cancer show wide ambivalence with some regarding screening as routine and responsible health behaviour and others seeing the test as exposing them to risk and uncertainty through diagnostic processes (Faulkner, 2012). There are clearly some parallels to be made with female attitudes to screening for and diagnosis of breast cancer discussed above.

The experience of prostate cancer and the various stages of treatment potentially pose challenges to many men's sense of masculine identity in terms of virility, energy and physical strength. Other aspects such as sporting activity and ability to work may also be affected. Broom (2010) argues that the cultural silence around the symptoms and impact of the disease have contributed to problematising men's help-seeking resulting in very variable treatment outcomes. The main treatment options currently available include surgery (radical prostatectomy), radiation therapy and hormone therapy – all of which have a number of possible adverse physical and psychological side effects that can negatively impact quality of life (Broom, 2010). The type of treatment offered is contingent upon the stage at which the disease is diagnosed but all, to a greater or lesser extent, are associated with concerns over continence, impotence and pain potentially threatening men's sense of identity and wellbeing.

Chapple and Ziebland's (2002) qualitative study of men's experience of prostate cancer explored the ways in which masculinity is compromised and re-negotiated through transitions in embodiment that materially is the site of social interaction. Their analytical and empirical focus is on the body as a "real fleshy entity" (Chapple and Ziebland, 2002: 822) that they contend is a fundamental feature of corporeal identity and experience, that is inextricably linked to 'being a man' and performing masculinity of whatever kind. They, therefore, challenge the singular primacy of the body as process and social construction that has come to be seen as central to gender theory and wider sociological theorising about the body. Findings from the study involving interviews with 52 men diagnosed with prostate cancer reveal a plethora of responses towards the disease and its treatment.

Initial help-seeking on presentation of symptoms appeared often to be delayed, with men commenting that they resisted seeing their doctor because of not wanting to appear weak and not 'macho'. Illness can seriously disrupt male status. Reactions to treatment for the disease centred on loss of bodily control. This involved permeated bodily boundaries (incontinence) and diarrhoea which made men more conscious that they could not take their bodies for granted. Associated loss of confidence and a heightened sense of spatial awareness in relation to accessibility to lavatories when away from home in public spaces, created anxiety and undermined their sense of masculine self-worth. Impotence and reduced libido were also key themes and one participant's comments highlight the impact of impotence on his masculine identity following hormone treatment. He says:

> I mean I feel that I've lost all masculinity, I'm not a man anymore. I mean I'm just not. I mean if I were walking along with my wife, very slowly these days, and somebody accosted her I would sort of run away. I have no masculinity left. (Chapple and Ziebland, 2002: 833).

Preoccupation with unfamiliar embodied experience was also a feature of a Swedish study that drew on interviews with men with prostate cancer, specifically to explore issues of sexuality post-diagnosis (Klaeson et al., 2012). Participants in the Swedish study mourned the loss of their sexuality, with this seen as threatening to their masculine identity.

For some men in Chapple and Ziebland's (2002) study, the effects of hormone treatment were visible; this was experienced as negatively transformed gender embodiment. Hot flushes, the development of breasts and increased body weight were described as compromising their sense of 'being a man', giving rise to feelings of worthlessness and loss of male role, particularly the husband role. The theme of embodied change and vulnerability was also present in Kelly's (2009) findings from research conducted with men diagnosed with progressive prostate cancer. The dominance of the hegemonic phallocentric model as central to sexual intimacy strongly influenced men's sense of their sexual selves. Masculinity may be largely socially constructed, but the experience of prostate cancer as recounted in Kelly's (2009) study does return us to the inescapable reality that bodily presentation is highly constitutive of what it means to be a man in our society.

Another cancer specific to men is testicular cancer that usually presents in one testicle. This cancer is now very treatable and, when only one testicle is affected, sexual function is usually maintained and the ability to father children preserved. Treatment usually involves surgical removal of the testicle with the procedure known as an orchidectomy that, when performed at the early stages of the disease, is now almost 100 per cent successful (Chapple and Ziebland, 2004). Unlike prostate cancer, testicular cancer has the highest incidence among younger men aged between 25 and 35 years. Despite the high rates of curative treatment for the disease, the physiological connection of the testicle to male reproduction and, thus, to embodied 'maleness', renders this male health problem as sensitive gendered terrain.

The issues of sensitivity and performed masculinity are drawn out in Chapple and Ziebland's (2004) article that explored the place of humour in men's accounts of their experience of having testicular cancer. Their research incorporated a focus on the ways in which humour mediated the lived experience of the disease including hiding embarrassment, managing emotions and self-presentation to friends, family and work colleagues. Avoiding taking things too seriously and sharing a joke are seen as highly valued by men – being 'one of the boys' is often accomplished through shared humour (Coates, 2003; Watts, 2007b).

Humour is also a device through which to demonstrate particular types of masculinity and this applies in the context of health as it does in other life circumstances. Using humour in the form of amusing anecdote offers a discursive vehicle through which to deflect attention away from potential vulnerable positioning as a cancer sufferer as well as vulnerability in other contexts. This diversionary device is a feature of male-only interaction that Coates (2003: 37) argues makes difficult or embarrassing stories (particularly those of self-disclosure), 'tellable'. Narrative construction performs important gender work and men and women are actively engaged in constructing and maintaining masculinity and femininity in their story-telling. For men, 'talking tough' is a feature of hegemonic masculinity (Connell, 1995), that prescribes norms of acceptable maleness. Whilst these norms may be culturally restrictive in allowing men to express their emotions and fears, they can function as useful impression management tools (Watts, 2008). Metaphorically, these hegemonic norms provide the 'mask' of tough masculinity whereby the concealment of all traces of vulnerability is enacted as an essential part of men's self-presentation. Coates (2003: 196) characterises the cultural restrictions on men's behaviour at the hand of hegemonic masculinity as "distortions". However, in the context of Chapple and Ziebland's (2004) analysis, humour as discursive response to testicular cancer may be a valuable distortion, enabling men to communicate about the disease through gendered norms that do not undermine their self-esteem and thereby support the maintenance of 'normative' male identity.

As in the case of treatment side effects in prostate cancer, issues of visibility also apply to testicular cancer. Drawing on the same study reported by Chapple and Ziebland (2004), Chapple and McPherson (2004) discuss the reasons why some men decide to have a testicular prosthesis and others reject the idea. Concerns about self-image and masculinity were pivotal in the decision-making process. In the period following surgery a number of men in the study came to realise that their sexual function was not impaired and, with this central to their masculine identity, could see no point in undergoing the medical procedure of having a prosthesis inserted. Safety and not wanting to have further invasive treatment were also reasons for electing not to have a prosthetic implant. Other participants, however, saw the issue of prosthetic implants in gendered aesthetic terms and, not wanting to feel 'lopsided', opted for the procedure. Being 'whole again' and 'looking normal' were significant for some men in the study, with this linked to having confidence to embark on new sexual relationships without having to explain why they had lost a testicle. For these men the potential for comfortable intimacy was important.

Processes of embodiment related to the experience of having testicular cancer are complex and operate on both a practical and cultural level. Threaded through men's accounts of diagnosis and treatment of the disease in both the articles discussed above, is the need to ensure that their masculinity is not compromised. There are different ways of 'being a man' and the limited talk about feelings and the imperative to avoid showing vulnerability means that the men in the study had to devote a lot of effort into keeping up a front to maintain, as much as possible, their innate sense of masculinity, defined principally through dissociation from emotionality.

## Conclusion

This chapter has introduced and discussed a number of women's and men's health issues, highlighting their gendered nature and the role of gendered cultural norms in shaping illness experience and medical responses. The case studies are illustrative of gender as a dynamic and contingent concept that operates through discourses, social practices and cultural processes embedded in organisations and policies. Health and illness are key sites for the 'doing' of gender and the making/unmaking of masculinity and femininity. This is not ideologically-free territory and at a time when gender relations are changing, it would be easy to overlook the powerful influence of ideology that continues to shape women and men's different health careers. Things are certainly changing, in terms of employment and educational achievement, of marriage and child-rearing such that relationships between men and women now incorporate a range of practices that challenge traditional assumptions about gender identity. Despite this, gendered ideologies about care giving and the nurturing of children persist, drawing on notions of compassion, empathy and emotion – all female gendered attributes. The dominance of this gendered ideology in framing both attitudes to and the practice of care is the key theme of the chapter that follows.

# Chapter 4
# Ideologies of Health, Care and Gender

## Introduction

Individual health and being healthy have long been associated with the absence of disease as discussed in Chapter 1. Health that is experienced at the level of ordinary bodily functioning has the quality of transparency – that is we tend not to notice it and this *invisible* quality of health was also highlighted in the opening chapter. 'Being well' is highly subjective and dependent on factors such as energy levels, sleep, diet etc and is characterised as a positive state, but one without a specific identity. Illness as bodily malfunction, on the other hand, is primarily ordered through the process of diagnosis and in that medical sense, usually has a categorised identity. Medical treatment, that restores bodily equilibrium through removing disease or illness has been conceptualised as an agent of health. Images of health are typically presented in terms of being active and fit and idealised in youthfulness and exercise in the form of disciplined bodies, with this applying to men and women in equal measure. Health-related terms such as vigour and fitness, for example, suggest that health that is more valuable is usually more than just the absence of disease or infirmity. Enhanced health carries various images of 'being active' that are the antithesis of 'sickness'.

This idealised notion of individual health has in recent years been extended to consideration of healthy (not dysfunctional) families and beyond to 'healthy communities' where the tasks of care and paid work, as part of a citizenship model, can be managed to optimise benefits for the individual, the family and the economy (Lister, 1997; Crompton, 2006). The opportunity for health, however, is complex situated as it is at the nexus of ethnicity, class and gender. The integration of these aspects within a social constructionist approach directs attention to competing gender displays across different arenas such as family, work and education and this is considered in Chapter 9 that has as its theme the topic of intersectionality. Whilst, as argued by Lewis (2014), health and caring for health are constituted through a combination of science, hope and hype, it is also the case that health and healthcare are shaped by persistent idealised notions of these constructs. In Western industrialised societies men and women have different health careers with roots in the gendered ideology of health and in wider gendered social relations. This chapter examines the way in which the ideological association of femaleness with caring, enacted through reproduction and dominant in the private sphere as part of family ideology, has become embedded in the public sphere with the majority of work directed at caring for health undertaken by women.

The term ideology has been defined in different ways according to context but can be broadly understood as the establishment of a set of values and beliefs that are usually culturally framed and defended. Ideology, as a pattern of meaning is contestable. Ideology that successfully establishes a pre-eminent way of thinking becomes a dominant ideology with hegemonic characteristics. Ideology may serve the interests of one group at the expense of another. The power of ideology to shape our attitudes, choices and actions through internalisation of particular values (that may run counter to our interests) is highlighted by Dalley (1996). Ideologies of care comprise a wide taxonomy including being 'other focused', compassionate, nurturing and patient, particularly in response to the needs of the young and the vulnerable. The family, as the principal site of care for the young, the elderly, those with disabilities and the infirm, has been the subject of extensive conceptual critique, particularly by the feminist lobby. Assumptions about the nature and structure of families and about the roles of men and women in family life have begun to be questioned but the gendered arrangements in mixed-gender families have remained largely unchanged. Although ideologies of both care and the family are entangled, their separate but related constructs merit closer scrutiny because of their gendered attributes that impact on health and healthcare work. Some of these ideas were touched upon in Chapter 2 but a more in depth articulation of the concept of the family and the consequent gendered relations of much care work is needed to more strongly situate the themes of later chapters, particularly working for health that is the topic of Chapter 5.

This chapter begins by discussing the idea of the *traditional* family with its huge cultural resonance that continues to influence normative assumptions about men's and women's care responsibilities across the life-course. Following consideration of the significant changes we have seen over the past century in women's engagement with paid work and the rise of different family forms, the discussion then moves to consider how care predicated on traditional family norms is conceptually and materially gendered. The final topic in the chapter concerns the critical issue of balancing the work ethic with the care ethic to contribute to health and welfare in their broadest sense. Ideas about breadwinning, nurture and interdependency are central to this 'balancing act' that for many women and some men is experienced as highly stressful with implications for mental health. The chapter closes by drawing out some key themes that will be revisited in later chapters.

## Social construction of the family

Family has been defined as a "heterosexual conjugal unit based on marriage and co-residence" existing mainly for the purposes of rearing children as well as the site for sexual companionship (Silva and Smart, 1999: 1). Traditionally family and marriage have been seen as protective and nurturing mechanisms – protective for women and children and nurturing for all family members with the *service* of providing nurture the responsibility of women. Above all, family and marriage have been idealised as a locus of care and also as a site for making gender distinctions. The recent gay marriage debate has, in part, been about whether marriage is an institution that is inherently gendered or whether it can be separated from the idea of a union between a man and a woman.

In historical terms marriage was often as much about establishing a site of power in the form of a political union as it was about romantic love (Ryle, 2012). With alliances, power, marriage, children and legacy inextricably interwoven, women were often the method or 'currency' of exchange in these power systems ordered by men. Coontz (2005: 42) makes this explicit, arguing that marriage alliances were not established between men and women but between men by *means* of women, thereby ensuring the control of women as part of the crucial cycle of reproduction and continuity of power. Love marriage is a fairly recent development. Ryle (2012: 323) comments on a further aspect of the politics of marriage, highlighting the 'marriage gradient' as a function of these systems, with women more commonly "marrying up" and men "marrying down" in social hierarchy terms. The extent to which, in some societies the institutions of family and marriage continue to be ordered through tribal rather than individual or personal interests, continues to engage anthropologists and other social commentators working in diverse cultural contexts.

Changes to the composition of families have been the focus of much media and scholarly attention for many years and in recent times have become a 'football' tossed around for political gain and ideological advantage by successive governments. The rise in cohabitation, separation, divorce, lone parenthood, step-families and the numbers of people living on their own has, in recent decades, led to significant changes in family relations and practices with the issue of a new family demography increasingly the subject of controversy and political debate (Williams, 2004). In contemporary Western society families come in a multiplicity of forms – single-parent families, foster families, same-sex families, re-formed families and single-person families are some examples of diverse family arrangements. Demographers identify a further trend in family forms – that of couples in long-term committed relationships not living together as a matter of choice; those in this group are called LATs, *living apart together* (Ryle, 2012). Particular family arrangements, such as those of some lesbian partners, may be an active rejection of traditional connotations of family and be a conscious decision to live outside the perceived confines of gendered family roles. Such choices may have been influenced by feminist thinking about heterosexual marriage that theorises marriage principally as a construct through which women are exploited and controlled by men (Barrett and McIntosh, 1982; Pateman, 1988). However, despite feminist warnings of this kind and the growing diversity in family structures, Gillies (2003: 2) signals caution in focusing too heavily on family change, arguing that statistical data "demonstrate an enduring continuity of traditional ties, with the majority of families still composed of a heterosexual couple".

Composition of and relationships within families comprise a many-layered picture and structural change within families interacts with other social changes to impact on experiences of family life. For example, the increased participation of young people in higher education together with a huge rise in housing costs have led to 'children' remaining for much longer in the parental home (*Guardian*, 15 April, 2009). This trend challenges in a material way the assumption that young adulthood is a period marked by increasing autonomy and independence from family ties. However, young adults are not and never have been a homogeneous grouping and the concepts of dependence and autonomy vary significantly between cultural groups (Gillies, 2000). In some cultures the transition to adulthood is characterised by developing greater responsibility for other family members rather than as a move towards individual independence (Gillies, 2000). Another example is the establishment of multicultural societies in many countries of the West such that care commitments may be a global issue stretching across continents. The experience of transnational families often involves some members relocating to higher wage economies principally to be able to help finance the family in their country of origin (Yeates, 2008). Although the plurality of family traditions now prevalent in Western society may be the source of greater gender equality (Holmes, 2009), the extent to which women are still expected to provide care for immediate and extended family members has its roots in family ideology centred on the assumed nature of women and the attributes required to care.

The postmodern family, as a changing and unsettled re-combination of family groupings fits much less comfortably into standardised categories than was the case in former times, even taking account of widespread extended family arrangements that have always existed. Disrupted norms of 'the family' have been seen by some traditionalists and moralists as posing a threat to the institution of the family with the ideological primacy of the nuclear family (see below) still a presumed norm. Family forms that deviate from this norm are often seen as a social problem, with a number of social policy initiatives directed at solving the issue of 'problem families' that may exhibit patterns of substance abuse, violence and incest. In public narratives this also has a strong class dimension, with intervention increasingly focused on finding solutions for patterns of working-class family socialisation labelled as 'troubled' and this associated with worklessness, delinquency, fecklessness, disorderly lifestyles and less than ideal parental role models (Dominelli, 2010).

In the UK context, strong 'hard working' families operating independently of state support have become idealised in political rhetoric that, until fairly recently, has consistently promoted the image of the male breadwinner and the family-focused (even if not entirely stay at home) wife/female partner as an idealised and 'proper' version of family, often termed as the nuclear family (see Hakim, 2006, for an extensive critique of women's home/work preference model). Central to the male breadwinner family model is an expectation of the man earning a family wage sufficient to sustain all family members – the ideal family wage has thus been perceived as a male wage. The concept of a wage is not a gender-neutral term but one that carries much historical baggage limiting women's involvement in paid work. Women's restricted participation in the labour market and consequent lack of autonomy are integral to the composition and practice of the nuclear family with a clear demarcation of power relations along productive and reproductive lines. In this model men are the producers of goods and services and women are the carers and reproducers of the family. This is the Parsonian ideal family structure and, though developed in the 1950s, this normalised version of what an ideal family looks like still has resonance today (Parsons and Bales, 1956). Culturally, we still hold men accountable for breadwinning and women for mothering, irrespective of whatever additional responsibilities they may have. Burnett et al. (2013: 632) add that: "organizational assumptions which frame fathers as breadwinners, ignoring their parental role, remain extraordinarily persistent because policies (no matter how long established) do not necessarily change social attitudes and behaviours".

Although this simplistic breadwinner/home maker family model may now seem somewhat outdated, particularly in light of the huge changes brought about by technology and the restructuring of the labour market, idealised family types are still called upon to be the agents of emotional support, the transmitters of cultural capital and the providers of care for the young, the elderly and the vulnerable. In trying to fulfil these social obligations, many families are under considerable strain particularly as increasingly both men and women are working and finding they have to balance the demands of paid work, family care and other citizenship roles. Positive images of family are associated with work, stability and beneficial intimate relations in the private sphere resulting in the family's minimal engagement with the public sphere in terms of support, regulation and intervention.

## Gendering care

In the context of change to and fluidity in family forms, the dominant association of family with care and nurture based on the sharing of resources and a set of mutual responsibilities and obligations, continues. Family is defined not by its form but principally by what it does. In sociological terms, family and family values remain focused on relations of care that encompass tasks ranging from housework to helping a family member to have a bath. Despite assertions to the contrary, the 'modern' family has not lost its function. Another continuing theme across a range of research studies is that the perception endures that women are more naturally inclined towards caring roles. Although increasing numbers of men are taking up roles as nurses, as carers and as care workers, women, particularly within families, shoulder the bulk of different types of care. The ideological association of femaleness with care persists on both a normative and material level and, through a conceptual lens, privileges care as disposition over care as practice, as compellingly theorised by Oakley (1972) in the early days of second-wave feminism. Feminist scholarship has led the way in drawing attention to the ideological processes which comprise care and locate women in the social role of carer. Mary Daly's (2002) work has been particularly influential in highlighting the important distinction between biological and social reproduction in the nuclear family and emphasised its significance for analyses of care.

Silva (1999) argues that foregrounding care as disposition romanticises care such as in the paradigmatic role of mothering, for example, and ideologically locates care in terms of individual emotional investment theorised through a number of gendered assumptions. However, focusing on care as practice rather than disposition, Silva (1999) argues, allows for a democratisation of care as a learned practice that has the potential to challenge patterns of established gender relations across all types of care tasks. Here the democratisation of care contributes to a redoing of gender (seen as attitudes and activities consistent with one's sex category) but, in so doing, does not violate the integrity of the self–other relationship within care practice. The issue of whether or not this call for a shift in the ideology of care towards care practice as a market activity, only preserves the *illusion* of caring (as disposition), forms part of the focus of the next chapter.

Care, as both disposition and practice, is a major theme of Gilligan's (1982) seminal monograph *In a Different Voice* that sought to draw critical attention to what she saw as dispositional differences between men and women in the conduct of human relationships. I introduced Gilligan's (1982) ideas in Chapter 2 in the context of the development of different feminisms as part of the second-wave feminist movement but here focus, not on the essentialist/constructionist schism through which her contribution is often analysed in the social psychology literature, but on her influential critique of what care is and means. It is at this level, that I see her ideas to be of most continuing relevance.

Gilligan's (1982) theory of moral development considers the different approaches of men and women to ethical dilemmas they may face and has as its basic precept that women are more likely to respond with an ethic of care approach whilst men are more inclined to adopt a justice focus. The ethic of care approach is framed by connectedness that emphasises the 'we' construct whereas the justice paradigm is more impersonal. Her assertion does not make universal or essentialist claims as she acknowledges that women can and do think in justice terms and men in caring terms. Her thesis rather draws out the greater propensity for women and men to behave in these ways – ways, of course that can be seen, not just as dichotomous, but also as complementary. This forms part of the sameness/difference debate that continues to command attention from academic commentators. Gilligan's (1982) thesis conflates two distinct issues: are men and women really the same or different (different voice) and whether men and women should be treated the same or different in the policy arena. Concerned not with practices but with ideology, the different voice debate rumbles on and feminists and other social commentators continue to invoke sameness/difference formulations as a way of framing issues being addressed, this despite a vision of dichotomous gender distinctions seen by some as justifying and reinforcing gender inequality.

Although contested, Gilligan's (1982) brand of cultural feminism – the view that men and women belong to different cultures and have different emotional orientations remains influential, not because of the answers she provides, but because of the questions she raises. Gilligan's (1982) analysis draws principally on three separate but connected qualitative studies conducted in the US. The first was a college student study that explored the issues of identity and moral development amongst a small cohort of female and male university students. The second study, involving 29 women who were in the early stages of pregnancy, was concerned with decision-making about abortion that was being considered by these women. Both studies posed questions to participants about moral conflicts in their lives and the hypotheses generated were further refined and explored in a larger third study that focused on rights and responsibilities. In the third study a sample of males and females matched for age, intelligence, education, occupation and social class at nine points across the life cycle contributed data on conceptions of self and morality, experiences of moral conflict and choice together with judgments about hypothetical moral dilemmas.

From the three empirical studies Gilligan (1982) found that women tended to define themselves through relationships with others whereas men were more autonomous and more inclined to a world view through which they were separate from others adopting a more strongly articulated 'I' stance. Because connectedness is understood to be more aligned with subjectivity and emotion, and justice more concerned with rights and prescriptions, male ways of decision-making have been seen as more robust or authoritative, particularly in the public sphere of politics and business. Reason rather than feeling is seen as easier to defend because of its supposed objectivity and detachment. In recent times, however, the so-called softer affective skills women may bring to business have begun to be more widely acknowledged though not necessarily more highly valued because they can be perceived to be an alternative to technical competence (Grugulis and Vincent, 2009; Hurrell et al., 2013).

Drawing on ideas from social psychology, Gilligan (1982) asserts that male ways of operating in the world have become normalised and in those terms the key issue women face in trying to become established in the world is that they are not men. In other words, the different attributes of women are less valued than those of men because they are judged according to a hierarchy of value that accords greater worth to male behaviour that is rooted in a long history of male power and control. In line with this history, modern societies have tried and, one might argue have been generally successful in, dividing men and women into different moral categories resulting in the gendering of care. In asking questions about men's and women's capacity for relational connection, Gilligan (1982) does not address diversity within the categories male and female because this was not part of her project. If she had been writing 20 or even 30 years later in an era of intersectional thinking becoming more dominant in sociological theory, this undoubtedly would have been different.

The key message we can take from Gilligan's (1982) thesis is that care is relational and as interaction involves being 'other-focused' that speaks to some measure of selflessness shaped by commitment to the other and attending to their needs. As so eloquently stated by Tadel (2014: 12), "the narrative of the 'other' contains the essence of how to care"; this also has temporal dimensions with Dykes (2006: 182) making the further claim that "caring time is cyclical and rhythmical allowing for relationality, sociality, mutuality and reciprocity". However, taking a group rather than an individual perspective, the notion of reciprocity (with care received and given across the life-course) ideologically positions care as both self-serving and other-serving. Recognition that self and other are equal serves to override the problematic tendency of the ethic of care to be idealised as *self-sacrificing* care in women's practices. The reciprocity of care model has not been in cultural ascendance so, although caring preserves both the group and the individual, it is the gendered relations of care developed through the institutions of marriage and family that shape dominant social expectations of *who* cares. Related to this, is the further question posed by feminist thinking that asks if women are socialised through gendered prescription to prioritise the care needs of others, how can they fulfil their needs and desires for their own care and wellbeing?

These aspects inevitably return us to consider in more depth what is understood by the term 'care', particularly as the word is an elusive concept used to describe a wide range of behaviours and tasks and it is also a word that is contested: the term 'being in care' is one example. We all develop our own personal ideas about caring and if we see behaviour that does not fit the mould, then we do not recognise it as caring. Care as warmth, protection and kindness in families is characterised by affection shaped by 'caring for', involving some element of 'doing' and 'caring about', centred on concern for another's welfare. Traditional gender roles in our society imply that men care *about* but women care *for*, with this distinction central to Gilligan's (1982) moral framework of care. Applying moral codes to care, either as disposition or practice, rather obscures what I see as the essence of care that is grounded more in the realm of necessity than in the realm of morality. Care as both affection and the undertaking of practical domestic tasks is central to the ideology of the family with most of the routine work of reproducing the family falling to women who are assigned the role of domestic specialist. The financing of families has historically fallen outside the care paradigm mainly because the activity of paid work usually takes place outside the home (this is changing with the rise of technologically enabled home working in many sectors). It could be argued, however, that resourcing families is integral to family welfare and, as such, is as much a care task as any other.

The term 'care' when used by professionals denotes some kind of work, usually paid work but not always, given the number of people who regularly volunteer in health and social care settings (see Watts, 2012). Care work has as a central feature looking after people and attending to their needs. Sulik (2007: 857) contends that: "care work is both gendered and relational defined typically as the care women do for others". Tasks such as feeding, changing bedding and attending to other physical and psychological needs all comprise care work. For those who receive care, the fact that they need this to help them function in daily life can lead to stigmatisation because care is often associated with dependence. In the case of infants and young children, dependence is seen as part of natural development towards competence and maturity and their care, usually situated within families, does not carry a negative label. Many of the tasks performed by paid care workers are also performed within families and it is not difficult to see how the boundary between formal (paid) and informal (unpaid and usually within families) care has become blurred. Because much of what we can describe as family care work is undertaken by women (irrespective of whether or not they are employed in a job), the female association with similar work in the paid labour market is difficult to dislodge. Clearly, although this association is neither universal nor inevitable, it continues to inform expectations about the practice of care across private and public spaces and attests to care as being engendered in both the market and private life. People's experiences of giving and receiving care are shaped, in large part, by cultural myths and stereotypes of gender which even decades of feminist theorising cannot dispel.

## Balancing acts and implications of gender for health

Work/life balance issues have been the subject of extensive commentary in literature on the sociology of work, with much of this having a focus on the dimensions of both family and gender. An important project for feminist politics has been exploring ways of reconciling the responsibilities of caring and earning. This tension, termed work/family conflict, is the lack of sufficient time in the day to meet work and family obligations. This time deficit has been exacerbated by an increase in work hours over recent years, especially for professional workers and for women (Blair-Loy, 2004). Traditional patterns of family life and modern patterns of female employment are not readily compatible.

In the contemporary corporate world 'ideal' workers who demonstrate high levels of organisational commitment are seen as those who can be responsive to employer demands and work long hours without the burden of family responsibilities. For the most part, they are typically male because work-devotion ideology reinforces the disconnection of work from other life roles and in most circles men are still revered and respected based on the kind of work they do. This ideology favours men over women, women without children over mothers and those who can afford to employ full-time care-givers over those with limited resources. It also disadvantages those who want to dedicate more time to parenting.

'Ideal' worker norms characterised by attachment to work at the expense of the rest of life have played an important part in highlighting particular issues faced by women in trying to balance the demands of paid work with family life. These demands can be excessive and Cha (2013) notes that mothers who work very long hours are more likely to exit the labour force entirely with this pattern more pronounced for those employed in male-dominated occupations. The norm of overwork in male-dominated workplaces and the gender beliefs operating in the family combine to reinforce gender segregation of the labour market. Obstacles faced by women in the workplace have come under extensive scrutiny and, in recent times, similar issues for working fathers have also received some attention such that increasingly scholars have begun to discuss work/life conflicts more generally in terms of parenthood. Postmodern notions of masculinity are more readily able to incorporate fathering practices and Coltrane (2008: 3) has argued that "it is now considered masculine to be a nurturing and involved father".

Against this background, the work of Gatrell (2005), writing about the sociology of parenthood, provides useful insights into changing family practices connected to the fulfilment of commitments to paid work and parenting. She presents a picture of the modern family as embattled and fragile and particularly the role of contemporary motherhood as conflicted and, on both an emotional and ideological level, almost 'undoable'. Hers is very much a middle-class perspective that highlights the practical and ideological demands on parents in their efforts to balance commitments to family and work – in this case mainly professional work. Her perspective specifically connects the idea of women 'having it all' to the public realm of work. Although the context of Gatrell's (2005) study that provides the empirical framework for her analysis is narrowly demarcated, the issues it debates have wider application beyond the book's immediate focus and it serves as a useful case study through which to explore how family ideology and care practices have changed.

The traditional male breadwinner/female home maker model of family life has been in significant decline for many years. A number of reasons for this are debated in the literature – changing social attitudes resulting in women's increased participation in higher education and the labour market, the exponential rise in housing costs requiring two incomes and the policy of successive governments advocating that mothers should be supported in returning to work to both fulfil their potential and contribute to the formal economy. The model of women being provided for by a male breadwinner has largely been replaced by dual income households as the norm, with women contributing to the family income as well as being able to have their own earned income. Financial resourcing of the family unit is now more commonly seen as the responsibility of both adults/parents whether in heterosexual or same-sex headed families. Women's paid work that was typically seen as an option, rather than a duty, has become more important in sustaining the family, even though men still generally earn more than their wives. Rigid notions of gendered caring do not fit well with most family experiences. A new ideology of the family has gradually emerged – one based notionally on practices that promote greater equality and, as noted above, this has become associated with the image of the modern woman 'having it all'. The reality, however, is more complex (Gatrell, 2005).

In former times, men's identification as sole breadwinners with the accompanying emphasis on the domestic sphere as women's domain gave rise to a clear division of labour between market work and domestic/care work. Dual income households disrupt this clarity and suggest a different set of shared responsibilities, one that crosses gender norms. I use the word 'suggest' because, as the critique that follows reveals, the rise of women's (including mothers of young children) participation in paid work has not been paralleled by a rise in the amount of domestic/care work undertaken by men. Whilst on one level women's claims to economic participation on equal terms with men have been recognised, women's relationship to the private sphere of the family seems to be little changed with this negatively impacting on their occupational status and career progress (Crompton, 2006). The phenomenon of the 'double shift' that refers to women working in paid roles and then carrying the major responsibility for domestic tasks has been widely reported. Its potential to negatively impact women's health, however, has received less attention.

Gatrell's (2005) critique of the institution of motherhood that Oakley (1976) argues grounds women's social position first and foremost in the family, captures both the biological and social constructionist perspectives that have been the focus of many commentaries. The ideal of women as home makers and nurturers of children, termed by Gatrell (2005: 45) as 'domestic goddesses', is explored in the contemporary context of many women having multiple roles. Social expectations of the good mother continue to have a strong temporal dimension with short quality time with children regarded by some as insufficient compensation for longer periods of absence away from them. The paradigm of the 'good enough' mother remains contested, particularly when contrasted with the selfless 'moral mother' celebrated in Gilligan's (1982) study that points to the ways in which selflessness is one of the conventions of femininity that continues to be structured by domesticity.

The further issue of maintaining the fabric of the home is, in part, a function of class – professional families may be able to employ a gardener, a cleaner and even a dog walker to ensure the smooth running of the home. Families in lower socio-economic groups are less likely to have this as an option. The employment of domestic help, whilst easing the domestic care burden, still has to be organised and managed and, as noted by Gatrell (2005), this can entail considerable emotional input from the person who is doing the contracting of the labour – this usually being the woman of the partnership.

Increasing longevity means that the care of both old and young family members falls to many families to organise and responsibility for this is often delegated to women, with potential negative implications for their health. A further factor in the responsibility matrix is that elucidated by Ugreninov (2013) who found that care for elderly parents is mainly provided by employed middle-aged women, many of whom are mothers of dependent children. Keeping everything running seamlessly and ensuring that the family's welfare is not undermined through mothers taking up paid employment, contributes to what Maushart (2002) terms as 'wifework'. Williams (2000) asks the question 'why are more intensive demands placed on women?' Is it that women are better time-managers or that they are more accommodating or just that they take the view that they cannot realistically share these tasks with their male partners? Maintaining some semblance of conventional gender expectations may be a way of husbands and wives retaining a sense of gender difference that is an important touchstone for constructing individual identities within the family. The literature provides no clear answers to these questions but the psychological strain caused by a number of competing household, life and work demands can be overwhelming (Watts, 2007c).

This chapter began with discussion of some of the ideals of being healthy such as keeping fit, eating sensibly and watching one's weight.

For many women (and some men) the pressure to *look good* and attend to details of appearance and adornment that is a daily presentation of self, can be experienced as stressful and add to the requirement to stretch the day even further. Working mothers, particularly those with professional careers, as members of the 'having it all' generation of women, cannot readily ignore the various demands of impression management in the workplace as they endeavour to be seen first and foremost as workers (see Watts, 2008 for more detail on this topic). Kumra and Vinnicombe (2010: 521) see the work of impression management as a function of what they describe as "impressing for success". They argue that women need to accumulate social capital in terms of networks and guidance, particularly gaining access to influential sponsors. Especially important for women is their conforming to masculine organisational cultures that they have had little say in creating; this can take considerable additional energy. Attention to these and other aspects of self presentation together with the need to constantly keep childcare arrangements operating smoothly as well as focusing on the intimacy of family relations can be experienced as very stressful and may impact negatively on mental health, with implications for gender. Commenting on the propensity for women to be labelled as mentally ill more often than men, Rogers and Pilgrim (2005) note that, women become more vulnerable to this labelling when they fail to conform to gender stereotypical roles as mothers, wives and carers. They make the further point that, although in historical terms the association of women and mental disorder is a relatively new phenomenon, professionals from a range of disciplines and lay people have sought to define mental illness in a feminised way (Rogers and Pilgrim, 2005: 71).

Freeman and Freeman (2013), in their text that investigates whether rates of psychological disorder are different for men and women, set out with great clarity what is currently known about gender and mental distress and also what, through rigorous analysis, we might reasonably claim or understand as causality in terms of women's and men's risk of suffering mental health problems. Mental health issues that most commonly centre on psychological and emotional problems are a global concern and, according to the World Health Organisation, constitute the number one cause of disability in the world. Ten to twenty per cent of people will experience depression at some point in their lives and women are more likely than men to develop the condition. Freeman and Freeman (2013) present data from 12 epidemiological surveys that attest to psychological differences between the sexes. However, the extent to which these differences are the result of biological factors or the product of social and cultural factors points to the pivotal issue of gender and mental health. The feminist lobby has made a significant contribution to the debate about gender and mental health arguing that psychological disorder is essentially a gender issue with high numbers of women traditionally treated for mental illness by the overwhelmingly male-dominated profession of psychiatry. Writing in the early phase of second-wave feminism, Broverman et al. (1970) were able to provide research evidence of gender bias in the construction of notions of mental health. Their research showed that behaviour defined as male was viewed by psychiatrists to be congruent with healthy behaviour, while behaviour defined as female was not.

In the analysis of the survey data in their study, Freeman and Freeman (2013) highlight that certain problems such as depression are more prevalent in women and others such as alcohol and substance misuse are more common in men. The old adage that women worry and men drink, though simplistic, appears to hold a kernel of truth. Overall, however, the 12 national surveys discussed by Freeman and Freeman (2013) point towards the conclusion that women are more likely than men to experience a mental health disorder. Explanations, though complex and multi-dimensional, will come as no surprise. In general, women appear to experience higher levels of mental distress because of the demands of role overload, specifically their social roles as home maker, carer and breadwinner. These competing roles can give rise to women feeling that they have 'failed' or not 'matched up' in one or more of these aspects with this experienced as negative self concept or low self-esteem making women particularly vulnerable to psychological disorders. Men also can experience role overload, but the expectations for men to combine employment and family care are less from both society and the family. Mental health problems are usually neither innate nor inevitable and Rogers and Pilgrim (2005) contend that it is the roles and context of people's situations that influence the type and rate of mental distress, rather than anything intrinsic about being a man or woman. Social pressures connected to gendered expectations and assumptions significantly shape the context of most people's lives. Freeman and Freeman (2013) thus argue that gender can no longer be assumed to be a marginal issue in considering the causes and treatment of mental illness.

## Conclusion

Embedded within notions of caring we can see some of the deepest dimensions of traditional gender differentiation in our society. Whilst the essentialist argument that women are nurturing and men are not is both overly simplistic and intellectually sloppy, it is the case that the social organisation of moral responsibility has expected women to seek personal fulfilment by caring for others and men to care for others by sharing the material rewards of independent achievement. Underlying these gendered arrangements are relations of symbolic power. A narrative has thus developed that talks of men caring about work, money and career advancement as externally validated sources of prestige and status contrasted with women's care for their families and friends and the 'doing' of the direct work of caring, often in domestic spaces. This social script that highlights idealised gender norms is highly simplistic and does not critically engage with the entangled understandings of care as a diverse form of labour. For example, women working in paid jobs to financially provide for their families are now often involved in 'caring about' tasks in ways that formerly were seen as the province of men. The meaning of care is increasingly ambiguous and new patterns of gender convergence are starting to emerge. However, because the *virtue* of care has been idealised as relational connection, the more instrumental nature of some caring tasks can result in them becoming marginalised across a spectrum of care 'worthyness' that is characterised by gendered meanings.

Feminist analyses of care have broadly accepted that the traditional narrative about caring and gender is more or less correct, both reinforcing and responding to persistent gender ideologies in the way we construct our public and private selves. Conflicts over how to resolve the basic tensions between family and work as well as reconciling strategies for the nurturing of self with commitment to others contribute to a long-term renegotiation of the gendered division of labour, opening up possibilities for a new politics of quality of life for both women and men. Changes to family structures and practices as well as to the labour market suggest that models of care may become less gender-bound and will need to respond to the wider challenges of changing demography, particularly the care demands associated with an ageing population. The implications of this for both men and women will be experienced at the familial level and also in the workplace where some of the gender demarcations connected to different types of healthcare roles are gradually being eroded. The subject of working for health is the theme of the next chapter that draws out the ways in which gender both shapes and reinforces expectations about the types of work women and men take up across the health and social care sector.

# Chapter 5
# Working for Health

## Introduction

The division of labour has been a longstanding preoccupation of sociology that has drawn out a number of analyses for various demarcations including those of professions, occupations, management and unwaged care-giving. The importance of class for sociology scholars in understanding the social organisation of work has always been of pre-eminent concern. More recent debates in sociology about the purpose, meaning and organisation of work across both public and private settings have been increasingly informed by gender as well as class dimensions, highlighting the cultural expectations of the types of work seen as suitable for women and men. Men as more suited than women to the 'heavy' work of construction, is one example of a work setting defined by gender (Watts, 2007a).

Work as a gendered construct has now been extensively theorised within work sociology discourses and a range of critical reflections on gender and work were introduced in the opening chapter. The social attributes of work have also been given prominence by a number of writers and these, contrasting with the utilitarian economic characteristics of work, direct attention to the importance of work in the creation of collective and individual identities (Allen and Pilnick, 2005). The entry of women in vast numbers into the labour market over recent decades has provided many women with an identity as worker beyond the identities of wife/partner and mother. This *female* worker identity has been further strengthened by the increased amount of time that many women are active within the labour market (Edwards and Wajcman, 2005).

The importance of the worker identity to women may explain why rates of work satisfaction among men and women are reported as higher for women despite their lower income earning capacity (see Palmer and Eveline, 2012). Bolton and Houlihan (2009) note, however, that high rates of job satisfaction among women are likely to be related to low rates of expectation. High status, well-paid jobs are seen as being beyond the reach of many women and they are thus satisfied with what they have. This is one rationale of the impact of a labour market divided by gender. Personal service workers, who are mainly women, derive meaning and satisfaction from their work via caring labour that is essentially 'people work' based on relational encounters (Bolton and Houlihan, 2009). Morgan et al. (2013) support this job satisfaction thesis in their exploration of rewards and job satisfaction in frontline healthcare work, often labelled as 'bad jobs' with low pay and few benefits. They found that workers derive significant intrinsic (for example, performing meaningful tasks) rewards from this work that requires a deeper level of relational connection with clients than other kinds of service work.

The concept of adaptive preferences (Colburn, 2011; Khader, 2011) offers an alternative explanatory framework for the satisfaction thesis discussed above. The concept, as outlined by Colburn (2011: 52), is "the unconscious altering of our preferences in light of the options we have available". Adaptation in this model is principally shaped by covert influences of which we are unaware. Khader (2011) specifically relates adaptive preference theory to women's oppression, arguing that a key feature is that women become accustomed to their oppressed circumstances and come to prefer them with this preference acting as a practical obstacle to changing them.

The link between macro-systems of work organisation within healthcare and the micro-level of individual workers' experience is explored below through the prism of gender. Issues of pay, career opportunities and occupational hierarchies and divisions between qualified and unqualified staff surface throughout the chapter with gender emerging as a pivotal influence on the structure of the health workforce in Western contexts. Changes to the way in which healthcare is both delivered and experienced have been driven by the introduction of new technologies and other scientific innovations producing equipment designed to perform medically complex tasks, bringing change to many areas of clinical practice. Discussion of these important developments and their impact on gender does not form part of this chapter, but is a central theme in Chapter 6 that follows.

For the current chapter, the focus is on different occupational and professional healthcare roles that have traditionally been the subject of gender demarcation but are currently undergoing considerable gender redefinition, at least at the level of practice if not in the public mind. The ideology and practice of nursing is first discussed followed by consideration of medicine and medical practice that historically has constituted a highly gendered form of professional 'boundary work' (Allen and Pilnick, 2005). This is slowly changing due, in part, to the growing focus on women's health that has its roots in feminist health advocacy, bringing an added demand to increase the number of women doctors in all fields (Riska, 2010a). An international trend has been the expansion of women's health centres that are dedicated spaces *for* women's health – run by women for women to improve women's health (Armstrong, 2010). Gender stratification in healthcare management is the third and final topic of the chapter. The rise of managerialism within healthcare in ways more familiar to business and industry than to care services has given rise to the features of market-based competition, performance indicators, audits, centrally-driven targets and other kinds of service evaluation and protocols. These measures, involving parameters such as league tables and star ratings, have quickly become associated with images of unnecessary bureaucracy and excessive 'red tape' and are seen by some as material obstacles to the delivery of healthcare and as an assault on the professions (Freidson, 2001).

Emerging from these initiatives is criticism of managerialist approaches that make the measure of performance more important than the impact of the performance itself. Rules designed as means to ends, have become ends in themselves, giving rise to the criticism that the health service is losing its customer focus (Sheaff, 2005). Some (see, as an example, Heubel, 2000), however, see the construction of patients as customers within a market-led healthcare system as problematic and incompatible with a justice model of healthcare. These administrative and management practices are not gender-neutral processes, and much critique of their operational value has failed to uncover how the emphasis on rationality and detachment within management practice is imbued with male gender bias with implications for individual career progression.

## Destabilising gender – the case of nursing?

Nursing is historically, culturally and ideologically female-dominated and there is now a well-developed literature on the gender relations of nursing and nursing practice that has been characterised as a form of feminised service work shaped by provider/client interaction, often requiring extensive amounts of emotion work (Simpson, 2009). Despite efforts to recruit from both the male and female population, the numbers of men entering the nursing profession remains low and men comprise just over 10 per cent of registered nurses in the UK (McLaughlin et al., 2010). The reasons that men might be reluctant to pursue a career in nursing range from the personal to the societal. Stokowski (2012) draws on evidence that suggests that men are induced to enrol in nursing careers during times of economic recession but seek jobs elsewhere in more 'male-appropriate' careers when the economy recovers. Another factor is attrition with males more likely than females to leave pre-registration nurse training programmes before completion. Although attrition is a complex issue involving diverse factors, McLaughlin et al. (2010) report that prevalent stereotypes and gender bias inherent in nurse education may make the experience of being a nursing student an uncomfortable one for males.

In Britain nursing became established in the mid-nineteenth century as an independent occupation for middle-class women with demonstration of a *caring attitude* seen as an essential attribute to take on the role of nurse (Davies, 2003). A *caring self*, discursively constructed as a normative feminine ideal with family care skills transferred to the care of patients, continues to position nursing as women's work. Other attributes of nursing involve following rules, being deferential to doctors and observing routines in monitoring the welfare of patients – elements of submission and reduced status contribute to these behaviours that are subject to the approval of powerful men, particularly male doctors and senior managers (Carpenter, 1993; Davies, 2003). However, the literature suggests that these normative behaviours as a function of the traditional inter-professional relationship between medicine and nursing are beginning to be renegotiated, with nurses using a number of strategies to resist medical dominance in the clinical encounter (Hughes, 2010). In practice nurses take on more decision-making responsibilities than their formal place in the clinical hierarchy allows, including diagnostic and treatment responsibilities. Where nurses are very experienced and are interacting with junior doctors, they may even end up telling the doctor what to do (Carmel and Baker-McClearn, 2012).

Because relations of domination are inherent in how medicine and nursing have been historically and culturally constructed in relation to each other, changes towards more collaborative inter-professional working is likely to remain at a slow pace. With this in mind, we also need to be aware that other social divisions impact on nursing's relation with doctors. Nursing is not comprised of a homogeneous set of interests and itself is internally divided along class, education and ethnicity lines as well as along gender lines. In addition, the demarcation between healthcare assistants (unqualified healthcare workers) and registered nurses (qualified professionals) has, in recent times become blurred due to some overlap in their roles and responsibilities in relation to care tasks (Mckenna et al., 2004). As a result concerns have arisen about the fluidity of job boundaries and, although nurses see healthcare assistants as having a subordinate role in the healthcare hierarchy, this fluidity could be a threat to nursing's professionalisation project that has been modelled on lines similar to those adopted for medicine (Bach et al., 2012).

With the move towards making nursing an all-graduate profession in the UK (for new entrants), we are likely to see the involvement of qualified nurses concentrated in the more technical aspects of complex care, with basic patient care (feeding, bathing etc) left to healthcare assistants that, as part of the nurse education reforms of the 1980s, have replaced the auxiliary nursing grade. This aligns with more recent intensive health sector reforms and the growth in lower status healthcare occupations that have reinforced occupational boundary disputes and given rise to workplace tensions between nurses and healthcare assistants (Bach et al., 2012). Healthcare assistants in Bach et al.'s (2012) study comment on the rewarding emotional connection they have with patients, suggesting that nurses would "do a better job" if they adopted a more down-to-earth approach in their interactions with patients, specifically emulating the behaviour of healthcare assistants. Lower pay and lack of training opportunities contribute to resentment on the part of healthcare assistants who, despite recognising their essential input to patient care, consider they are a marginalised group of workers within the healthcare hierarchy.

Registration as a qualified nurse in the UK is the successful culmination of a prescribed university programme of theoretical study and supervised practice learning designed to prepare students for employment in a professional clinical role, usually within the NHS. A greater emphasis on academic learning now shapes pre-registration nurse education, contrasted with the former practice-based apprentice model of training based largely in hospital wards. Nurses are the largest group of workers with formal qualifications in healthcare and, once qualified, are increasingly aligned with particular areas of clinical expertise (Wrede, 2010; Carmel and Baker-McClearn, 2012). Specialisation within clinical practice, perceived as evidence of disciplinary maturity, has become culturally associated with excellence; this applies to nursing as it does to medicine.

The primary goal of nursing is to assist individuals towards activities that contribute to the recovery of health and independence; it is person-centred rather than disease-focused and 'good' nursing has the 'whole' person at its core. It is holistic in nature and values led. Whilst nursing cannot readily aspire to the socially elevated status of medicine, its contribution can be demarcated through the activities of practical and emotional support of patients and their families, often involving significant emotion work focused on the achievement and maintenance of independence (Hochschild, 1979). This kind of labour has been theorised on a number of levels but, in the case of nursing, involves assessing patients' needs and responding to them appropriately and establishing an emotional connection with the patient. Nursing practice is based on a relationship between the nurse as worker and the patient as care recipient and as such is a form of relational service work (Cranford and Miller, 2013). Nurses managing their own emotions in the interests of patient welfare contribute to good care involving a combination of organisational skills, physical labour and emotional labour. These are the key components of frontline nursing practice where all nurses begin their career and it is the relational elements that are often accorded the label 'real nursing'.

Relational aspects are particularly to the fore in some specialist areas of nursing practice such as gynaecology that is the focus of an insightful commentary by Bolton (2007). She considers how women construct and celebrate their status in carrying out what can be seen as the stigmatised 'dirty work' of nursing connected to the dissolution and failure of women's bodies. This morally and physically tainted area of nursing is characterised by Bolton (2007) as essentially a woman's world, with women nursing women who are experiencing uniquely 'women's' problems. Socially difficult issues such as miscarriage, infertility, foetal abnormality and pregnancy termination are the materiality of this world. Bolton (2007) argues from her research data that this distinctive area of nursing practice is shaped by the 'doing' of gender. Her participants claim that only they as women are able to nurse the gynaecology patient proficiently, with this achieved through shared meanings drawn principally from their understanding as mothers. Whilst the nurses in Bolton's (2007) study were confident in their skills to provide sensitive and healing support to the women in their care, they were also acutely aware of their lesser status in relation to both midwives and junior doctors, the two groups of healthcare professionals with whom they had most contact. These reflections from this particular nursing community attest to the hierarchical and highly structured divisions within healthcare.

Despite nurses continuing to work in the shadow of medicine, not least because of nurses' more limited educational preparation, nursing has changed in many ways – it is now more professionalised with a stronger emphasis on academic educational components than was hitherto the case, facilitating higher levels of specialist expertise and more clearly defined and diverse career pathways. Opportunities to advance to senior positions in roles such as clinical nurse specialists or nurse consultant posts have enhanced career paths within nursing that has in recent years set out to promote its image as one of high academic attainment coupled with strong professional credibility. A variety of management, research and teaching posts are open to nurses who want to develop their careers beyond frontline care. Postgraduate qualifications in a range of nursing topics are now widely available and, for those nurses who seek to move into roles as clinical educators, such qualifications are a pre-requisite for appointment to higher education teaching posts.

A further change has been the move towards a more technically-centred model of practice within healthcare that has led to the emergence of a new kind of nurse, one as more of a physician's assistant that Carpenter (1993) argues has led to an internal division of labour within nursing. Some have characterised this development as potentially undermining of the 'softer' skills associated with the traditional craft skills of nursing and bedside care and encroaching on elements of the medical role (Davies, 1995). These 'soft' skills remain at the centre of the dominant vision of nursing, at least at the level of ideology. A sense that these skills are less valued in the professionalism stakes, has contributed to the recent debate about perceived poorer standards of nursing care, particularly on hospital wards.

Nurses' pay has also increased and for senior nurses in the UK, pay is on a par with that for long-serving teachers and lower/middle manager public sector workers. Increased financial rewards for nurses underpin an emerging interconnected global care chain with a growing flow of nurses from low-income to high-income countries (Wrede, 2010). Nurse education in some low-income countries, such as for example in the Philippines, has been tailored according to Western standards (Wrede, 2010). Another change has been to the gender composition of the nursing workforce, with slowly increasing numbers of male nurses entering clinical practice. Whilst the proportion of registered male nurses in the UK stands at only around 10 per cent of the total, their work in this professional role characterised by one male nurse as "not a normal male career" (Halford et al., 1997: 178), has been the subject of a number of commentaries. Writing on the topic has highlighted how men in 'female' roles such as nursing, by both disrupting and reinforcing traditional gender norms develop new practices to reshape power relations across gender boundaries. The work of Ruth Simpson (2009) is particularly insightful in this area and her case study of the ways in which male nurses deal with conventional notions of masculinity and femininity as gender transgressors is discussed below in terms of a reworking of gender rather than gender transformation.

In the context of nursing, Simpson's (2009) research explored how men see women and how women see men in their work roles, particularly in relation to the skills and attributes that each gender brings to the job and their performance as care-givers. Her findings, that draw on the Bourdieusian theoretical construct habitus, referring to the ways in which individuals find their place in the world and develop congruent dispositions and behaviours, set out examples of the sameness/difference gender discourse theorised by Gilligan (1982) and discussed in the previous chapter.

Simpson (2009) reports the views of female nurses about their male nurse colleagues in relation to several themes that include professionalism, breadwinning, career focus and caring capabilities. Women welcomed men as colleagues as they saw this as a trend towards greater levels of professionalism in nursing, particularly as it was recognised that men tended to gravitate towards management and education roles away from 'hands-on' traditional nursing care. Speedier male career progress was seen not to be at women's expense but was justified by appealing to breadwinner discourses as one woman comments: "men can often end up by being the primary breadwinner – if only for a time – I don't necessarily begrudge them it" (Simpson, 2009: 152). Men's reluctance to engage in the 'hard slog' of nursing care, described by some participants in Simpson's (2009) study as 'drudgery' and 'mind-numbing', was acknowledged thus: "it's quite a rare bird a male nurse as far as caring capabilities" (Simpson, 2009: 152). The issue of intimate care is sensitive and male nurses touching female patients in delivering intimate care may make them vulnerable to claims of inappropriate physical contact.

Men were seen as more suited to roles that involved them in technological aspects of nursing such as diagnostics and also in the more fast-moving arena of accident and emergency where they might have to deal with difficult and aggressive patients (Simpson, 2009: 101). These roles helped to remove men from association with the more routine and subservient aspects of nursing such as day-to-day bodily care of patients. Men were seen to provide balance to an otherwise all-female group that was perceived as potentially dysfunctional; their perceived greater incisive decision-making attributes were also valued, particularly in stressful situations when "things had gone wrong" (Simpson, 2009: 153).

An overarching perception of men by women in Simpson's (2009) research was their authoritative presence seen as "getting to the core of the issue" and not becoming emotionally involved. The issue of uncertainty in respect of what can be achieved for patients in terms of restoring them to health was highlighted as often problematic, with men more likely to know what to do for the best. Women's reflections on the presence of men in culturally feminised roles drew heavily on traditional notions of masculinity and femininity and seemed to support existing gender power relations. Wingfield (2014) comments that professions dominated by women are frequently low in salary and status and the entry of men in greater numbers may improve both prestige and pay. Men in Simpson's (2009: 152) study were on the whole warmly welcomed by female colleagues in a collegial work environment. Wingfield (2014: 369), also writing in the context of nursing, argues that: "building strong relationships with colleagues and supervisors often happens relatively easily for men in women's professions and pays off in their occupational advancement".

Men's comments about gender issues in the context of nursing highlighted other features of difference related to the cultural privileges of masculinity. They recognised that male nurses were treated less dismissively by doctors and their opinions were more likely to be listened to. This advantage was explained by culture, with women seen to be conditioned to accept their gender disadvantage. More widely, there has been an attempt by senior managers to reduce the importance of occupational boundaries in healthcare (Timmons and East, 2011) and the male nurses' perceptions that they were more readily heard by doctors might also be related to moves towards greater egalitarian status amongst healthcare professionals as a function of the disruption to traditional hierarchies discussed earlier in this chapter. Other advantages that can accrue to male nurses are those identified by Wingfield (2014) in respect of their interactions with patients, doctors and other staff who do not expect to see men doing a 'woman's job'. Sometimes this assumption means that male nurses are mistaken for doctors and ultimately contributes to a sense that they are more suited to the less 'hands-on' aspects of the role and are granted more authority and responsibility than their female counterparts.

Some men in Simpson's (2009: 155) study were critical of female colleagues describing them as emotional, less able to make quick decisions and more oriented towards the routine task system of work organisation (injections, giving medication, changing dressings and so on) rather than having a more holistic overview of patient care. Other men, however, spoke positively about their own capacity for emotional engagement acknowledging what they saw as their 'feminine side'. As one man commented: "the actual essence of nursing is to nourish, to nurture and I think that's instinctively a female thing … so I think as a nurse is thinking as a woman" (Simpson, 2009: 156).

Men's entry into nursing, as evidenced by Simpson's (2009) research, unsettles some aspects of gender relations but reinforces others. Simpson's (2009) data, richly descriptive in qualitative depth, presents extensive reflexive accounts of both male and female perceptions of entrenched assumptions concerning gender-appropriate behaviour within nursing that highlight how gender relations are embedded both within nursing and more widely in the organisation of paid work generally. The gender of a female nurse is unremarkable whereas a man found in this role is not just a nurse but a 'male nurse' (McLaughlin et al., 2010). Despite this increased visibility, it seems that norms of masculinity for male nurses are not in fact disrupted because of their greater access to arenas such as management largely removed from direct clinical practice, with this evidenced by their disproportionate representation in higher grades and management posts in what remains a female-dominated area of employment (Whittock et al., 2002). This aspect is further supported by Halford et al. (1997: 128) who comment on the "'male takeover' of the new nursing hierarchy". Significantly fewer male nurses than female nurses take up part-time employment that continues to be feminised across all employment sectors and viewed with suspicion in relation to part-time workers' perceived lower level of commitment to their careers, particularly in terms of their investment in skill development (Hakim, 2006). Men's reduced level of engagement in part-time nursing work may also account for men being able to advance their careers more rapidly than women (Whittock et al., 2002; Brown and Jones, 2004).

## Medicine, medics and the clinical gaze

Along with the law and the upper echelons of academia, medicine has long been perceived as an elite profession characterised by very strict entry criteria. Most professions have a system of registration and regulation which acts as a licence to practice, with this overseen by some form of governing body that admits to its ranks those who fulfil the entry criteria, excluding those who do not. These criteria, serving as protection mechanisms, delineate and defend professional boundaries. Abbott (1988), whose work on the sociology of professions remains a seminal text, refers to these bodies of expert knowledge as professional jurisdictions whereby both the culture and structure of a profession as an applied discipline, are created and maintained. Codes of conduct, education programmes, licensing of professional practice, regimes of accountability and requirements for the demonstration of continuing professional development all underpin professions that are shaped by powerful subcultures, with some carrying particular stereotypes. One example that draws on some of my earlier work is civil engineering that is closely associated with the construction sector characterised by the building site imagery of dirty and heavy physical working conditions (Watts, 2007a).

Professionalising movements have been crucial to the development of health occupations (Pascall, 1997) and, following the establishment of the NHS, medicine in the UK has become primarily a public sector profession, though many hospital doctors undertake private work that can substantially increase their income (Crompton and Lyonette, 2011). General practitioners (GPs) in primary care are self-employed and operate as small businesses with their income derived from public funds via NHS budgets. Changes to GP contracts have meant that they have been able to regularise their working hours by opting out of on-call and weekend working resulting in them working on average fewer hours than their hospital-based counterparts. Some consultants work very long hours because of private practice that can be extremely lucrative. General practice may be regarded as less prestigious but it is almost as highly paid as hospital medicine, with the average GP salary now in excess of £100,000 (Crompton and Lyonette, 2011). Medicine, in whatever form, is a highly paid profession.

As noted above, nursing – now incorporated as a graduate profession – carries the gender stereotype that positions women as more suited to enter its ranks. Medicine, too, has maintained its gender stereotypical image and its gendered scientific knowledge base that are both seen to be male, despite equal numbers of men and women gaining places at medical school. Women doctors are encouraged to focus on community and primary care (seen as a more family friendly but clinically inferior practice domain) rather than the high status specialisms such as surgery and medical research (Riska, 1993; Riska, 2010a). The status of women in the medical profession is still not on a par with that of men because medicine is internally segregated by sex; more female than male doctors work part-time and this is seen as seriously career-limiting (Crompton and Lyonette, 2011). Wallace (2014) highlights what she sees as the ambivalent status of female physicians who, on the one hand are present in increasing numbers but, on the other, are not fully socially integrated into medicine, receiving less instrumental support and sponsorship than their male colleagues. They do, however, according to Wallace (2014), experience more empathetic support than male doctors but the reason for this is uncertain. Wallace (2014) posits that this may be because women more actively seek this kind of support than men. Other recent research by Walsh (2013) that explored factors relating to the work/life interface affecting the wellbeing of doctors, reports the intensive work pressure and long hours as dominant features of the medical profession, especially in the hospital setting. She found that, although female doctors were more likely to experience job burnout than male doctors, they were less likely to leave their job because of being able to draw on greater levels of social support, particularly from family and friends.

Historically, writing about medicine and doctors has presented these in gender-blind terms, documenting how the practice of medical education is located outside the social processes of gender, race and ethnicity (Riska, 2010a). Throughout the nineteenth and much of the twentieth centuries, medicine was overwhelmingly male and early feminists, as part of extensive sociological scholarship, highlighted the generally gendered nature of doctors' attitudes and behaviour and the related exclusion of women from the most senior posts in the medical profession (Lorber, 1984). However, the changing gender composition of the profession and the call for more women doctors across all specialties, have given rise to a number of questions. Is medicine practised differently by women and men physicians? Will a greater number of female doctors bring a positive impact to women's health issues? The answers to these questions are ambivalent but some research such as that by Bertakis and Azari (2007) reports that, although female doctors use a more empathetic communication style with their patients, there are no other clear differences in the practice of medicine between men and women.

Increased longevity, generally better living conditions for most people in Western societies and advances in medical research have resulted in expectations for improved health across the life-course, with this seen as a human right. We expect doctors to be able to classify and then effectively treat our ailments. Drawing on the biomedical model, cure rather than care has become the goal of modern medicine that sees death as failure. Medicine, as an instrument of both individual and public health, has in recent years come under much scrutiny in terms of outcomes, competence, malpractice claims and justice related to distribution of scarce resources and the unequal access to healthcare services. No longer is medical care regarded as something for which we should be grateful but rather as something to which we are entitled and this as a function of the consumer movement for health and other social 'goods'. The practice of medicine is a mixture of rigorous science and uncertain indicators; as a system of knowledge, however, it has its own coherency based on activities of disciplined enquiry and investigation. Understanding of these processes that in part are rooted in both the history and philosophy of medicine has been theorised from a number of perspectives.

The ideas of Michel Foucault (1973) have been particularly influential in drawing attention to the development of the medical profession in ways that separate the patient's body from the patient's person or identity. This body/person separation, termed by Foucault as the 'clinical gaze', has made possible the analysis of the body as a site of competing power interests and has also positioned the body as an object for manipulation. According to Foucault (1973), pre-eminent power is invested in doctors through their investigation of bodily symptoms, disease diagnosis and treatment recommendations – all contributing to the 'legitimate' management and surveillance of both sick and healthy bodies within the paradigm of modern medicine that Armstrong (2001) argues has made us subject to an extended clinical gaze. Feminist work in medical sociology has emphasised how the clinical gaze has a gendered dimension with women's bodies more susceptible than men's bodies to surveillance through processes such as childbirth, premenstrual syndrome and menopause, with these experiences in a woman's reproductive life perceived not as natural stages but as illness within medicalised discourses (Bell and Figert, 2010; Nosek et al., 2012). Although women perceive menopause as a medical event, it is the social status passage of menopause that is emphasised by them as important (Ballard et al., 2001). Foucault's ideas are complex and challenging in equal measure and now are incorporated within medical education curricula to inform thinking about how bodily status in terms of function and deficits has gained precedence in the medical lexicon.

In former times, medicine and medical science, seen as disciplines detached from the humanities and social sciences, were less accountable for their practice. However, medicine is no longer just an 'intimate' private matter involving only the small circle of patient, family and physician. Now medicine is part of a wider arena where there are many witnesses and participants with multiple interests (Schneiderman and Jecker, 2011). In the digital age, 'tweets' and 'posts' can hold hospitals and doctors to account and social media have become a compelling force in health. The internet has transformed patients into mobile and effective influencers when formerly they were less informed and, as a result, more likely to be the passive recipients of services. Increasingly patients as health consumers are able to rate the quality of the services they receive and the associated prevailing discourse is that public pressure drives up standards with the resulting marginalisation of poorly performing clinicians and hospitals.

Stronger public engagement with medicine has resulted in its gradual democratisation (see Chapter 1) and the importance of interdisciplinary collaboration between medical research, epidemiology, clinical practice and the human and social sciences is now acknowledged (Lagro-Janssen, 2010). This aside, medicine is a multi-faceted business involving education, research and pharmaceutical components together with large-scale 'marketised' healthcare systems focused on frontline delivery of services. The concept of the internal market for health (principally between local health trusts as well as the purchaser/provider split) became a dominant organising principle within healthcare delivery in the UK during the 1990s. This contributed to medicine becoming highly politicised and variously used to serve the power interests of all parties across the political spectrum. At medicine's core, however, are the key processes of disease prevention and diagnosis, treatment that wherever possible is focused on cure and the maintenance of life, with this aspect increasingly reliant on specialist instrumentation and technological innovation that in many areas is developing at a rapid pace.

The complexity of large-scale healthcare systems, ordered through public and private organisations, consultation groups, different professional and regulatory bodies as well as government departments, has led to an increased focus within healthcare on all types and levels of management that now in the UK is strongly associated with a culture of managerialism. This culture, seen by some as compromising the principle of professional autonomy, one of the founding principles of the NHS and so fiercely protected by the medical profession, is shaped by consumerist drivers as well as the politics of technocratic change that Sheaff (2005: 188) argues is underpinned by the "ideology of efficiency". Some, in a more cynical tone, have voiced the view that the increased demands of managers are actually stopping health professionals from getting on with their job (Sheaff, 2005).

## Managing health

The part played by management in the organisation and delivery of healthcare, at both the strategic and local level, has come under much scrutiny by successive UK governments. Re-structuring of provision for primary and secondary care is part of a constantly changing environment for health within the NHS. Devolved responsibility to GPs for primary care budgets and the emergence of foundation hospital trusts are just two examples of recent change initiatives promoted on the basis of recognising and advancing 'best' expertise in particular aspects of healthcare delivery. We are told that change is needed to address the complex and often competing needs of service users, healthcare workers and senior managers. Negotiating the contradictions and tensions arising from these competing interests in a fast-changing context is at the heart of contemporary healthcare management. In parallel, the measurement of performance of the nurse, the doctor and other health professionals according to external yardsticks of impersonal and objective criteria, shaped by notions of evidence and targets, contributes to a plethora of mechanisms for managing performance (Barry et al., 2010).

Pre-eminent in the current change discourse is the issue of culture change specifically directed at making high quality personalised care that respects individual dignity, the number one priority. Managers are at the front line of innovation and change in healthcare and are the gatekeepers of the values of trust and inclusion seen as essential to good outcomes for patients. There is a legal duty on managers and their organisations within the NHS to provide healthcare services, with an increasing emphasis on practice-led management – the move to GP fund holding first introduced in 1991 is one example of the application of this concept. Although services continue to be structured around specialist groupings such as mental health, learning disability or older people, there is greater awareness of the importance of responsive service provision that connects across the multiple needs of service users – this almost as a form of 'service intersectionality'.

Managing health in a variety of roles is qualitatively different from managing in other contexts. Although the ideology of healthcare has, in recent times, come to incorporate features of the market model, healthcare as a service has distinguishing features from other kinds of services such as, for example, banking or insurance. People accessing healthcare have particular needs and many have limited choice regarding how and where they are treated. They may be stressed and they may feel unwell and be experiencing significant transitions in their lives. Management in this sector, it could be argued, more than in any other context, is a relational task because of the inherent vulnerability of those seeking care. Understanding of leadership as a relational practice, rather than as a heroic-individualistic performance, has been developed by Binns (2008) who focuses on the ethical implications arising from the pressures on leaders to instrumentalise and masculinise their relational work. She emphasises how reflexive practice that enables leaders/managers to understand the effects of their conduct on others can be an agent for transforming workplace relations. In the case of her particular study, Binns (2008) focused on the ways in which an ethical subject is a gendered construct through the lens of masculinised certainty and feminised self-doubt. The work of other writers such as Carli and Eagly (2007) theorises relational leading as a more democratic and participatory model and one more likely to be adopted by women.

Managing staff, budgets, work schedules, safety in the care environment as well as the challenges of inter-professional working are some of the concerns of the healthcare manager. Additionally in recent years healthcare management has been tasked with giving a greater voice to service users in the design and delivery of care (Martin and Finn, 2011). A further development has been efforts to increase the leadership capacity of healthcare professionals, particularly amongst lower-status staff without formal managerial power, with the creation of frontline leaders seen as a way of improving the quality of healthcare (Martin and Waring, 2013: 358). This initiative has faced considerable challenges and has had limited success due to entrenched structures in healthcare organisations that do not readily foster recognition of the potentially transformational nature of some frontline management roles (Martin and Waring, 2013). Traditional healthcare occupational hierarchies are characterised principally by clinical skill development rather than by training in leadership and management. In the complex organisational matrix of the NHS being a healthcare manager is multi-faceted, with specific challenges that are not part of mainstream corporate management; management in this professional context has become very heterogeneous.

One particular challenge identified by Bolton (2005: 5) concerns managing health professionals that she argues has been "enduringly problematic" because of their reluctance to comply with management edicts that could compromise their self-governing clinical authority. One solution posited by Bolton (2005) and by Martin and Waring (2013) has been to 'recreate' health professionals as managers. Bolton's (2005) study that focused on nursing roles revealed how senior nurses were keen to embrace the management function, but only within the comfort of existing hierarchical structures. The opportunity to have a management rather than a clinical career in healthcare is seen by some as an attractive and, possibly, a more lucrative option, particularly for nurses in terms of their upward social mobility. Clearly, different levels of management responsibility involve different demands and offer different rewards. However, we know from recurring media reports that, although managing in healthcare always operates against a background of financial restriction, many NHS managers in senior executive roles are very highly paid with this justified by excessive work demands due to the dynamic nature of managerial change (Barry et al., 2010).

The issue of the gender composition of healthcare management has received limited critical attention in recent scholarship, but can be explored against a background of the now well-documented critique of problems facing women in a wide variety of management roles. Despite the large increase in the numbers of women entering the labour market in recent years (Burke and Nelson, 2002), they remain under-represented in corporate leadership roles (Vinnicombe and Singh, 2002). Management is associated with masculine behaviours that involve competitiveness, instrumentality and individuality (Barry et al., 2010). A wide literature on the gendered relations of management has developed that suggests that, although equal opportunity and affirmative action are now embedded within the corporate recruitment strategy of many organisations, women are still unable to rise to top management posts in significant numbers. Due Billing (2011: 298) notes that "managerial jobs have conventionally been understood as male and thus as not being directly suitable for women". This perception reflects and produces a variety of barriers that create a glass ceiling effect (Cook and Glass, 2014).

Drawing on findings from an international comparative leadership study across 27 industrial nations, Moore (2014) reports that compared to men, women in senior management roles are less likely to be married and also to be parents. Those who do have family responsibilities, however, spend disproportionately more time on household labour than their husbands. Moore (2014) also reports that 70 per cent of the senior male managers in her study had female partners who were not in employment or were working in non-professional jobs with no supervisory responsibilities. They were thus more available for childcare and housework and were able to have greater involvement in helping to build their husband's career that *ideally* should function unhampered by non-work demands. As noted by Blair-Loy (2004) and discussed in the previous chapter, the ideal career, especially among managerial elites, proceeds without interruption from its inception and is typically male.

Management, as a set of practices and behaviours, is heavily shaped by temporal aspects that Collinson and Collinson (2004: 240) critique in relation to the power of 'organisational time discipline'. They argue that this has contributed to a 'remasculinization' of management in which women managers at all levels will only survive if they follow the example of their male counterparts to subordinate home and family to company and career. It may be this aspect, more than any other that can make the managerial identity hard for women to bear (Barry et al., 2010). Powell (1999) adds the dimension of demography, arguing that with falling birth rates, there are fewer candidates for managerial jobs with the balance shifting towards more women who want to work and fewer men available for work. Accordingly we are left with the question of why there are still so few women in executive management posts that carry 'clout' (defined by Burke and Nelson, 2002 as policy-making power). Exploring the alleged feminsation of management, Muzio and Bolton (2006) were led to a contrary position, concluding that management remains a male occupational project.

There are very few reported studies that explore the role of gender in relation to managerial behaviour within the NHS. Some work has focused on the impact of gender amongst senior nurses and nurse managers particularly the over-representation of men in senior nurse roles and this is discussed further below. Wider management structures within the NHS have had limited coverage in the literature and the ways in which gender might shape how management is 'done' remain an under-explored area. The study by Greener (2007) that examined interactions between senior male and senior female managers and between senior male doctors in the

NHS has been an attempt to bring gender centre stage in the analysis of management behaviour in this sector.

The background for Greener's (2007) study is the long-standing issue of the managerial class perceived as challenging the pre-eminent professional status of the medical profession, with the allied prospect of far-reaching reforms to NHS management structures. The relationship between doctors and managers is an extremely high profile one and health commentators ceaselessly assess changes to the balance of power between the groups. The balance of power, seen as being at the root of interactional difficulties between the two groups, has shifted in favour of managers but openly claiming this in the public arena is sensitive and, sometimes, counter-productive (Greener, 2007). Impression management, as a tool with which to play different roles as part of negotiation and discussion of potentially contentious issues, was the backdrop to Greener's (2007) analysis. He found that male managers focused on 'winning' encounters with senior medical figures, whereas female managers were more concerned with getting the job done and this held greater potential for a more inclusive approach, trying to 'carry' clinicians with them in the decision-making process. Greener's (2007) qualitative study is small-scale and uses a number of inter-related theoretical concepts to interpret his data. I am only capturing the key headline findings, but these are broadly consistent with other work on gender and managerial style, including that of Carli and Eagly (2007) introduced earlier in the chapter.

Nursing, as a route into healthcare management, has been the subject of a number of studies and the work of Brown and Jones (2004) draws out key factors to explain the place of gender in nursing hierarchies. Their study discusses gender segmentation within nursing. Gender segmentation arises when one gender is disproportionately represented in senior roles within an occupation. Segmentation of this kind has traditionally been explained by human capital theory, this being the sum of an individual's skills, qualifications, work experience and also, Brown and Jones (2004) argue, geographical mobility. Women spending less time than men in the paid labour force may reduce their experience and skills, so human capital theory might be a reason for their poorer occupational outcomes. Women and men often have different career histories, with many women taking time out from work to have a family and/or working reduced hours to balance work and caring responsibilities.

Taking the context of the nursing profession and using quantitative methods, Brown and Jones (2004) set out to test whether human capital was rewarded differently for men and women. Their findings show that qualifications, having taken up a previous senior role and working full-time with no career breaks since registration, were significant predictors of seniority in nursing. Length of nursing experience was not a predictor of seniority. Overall, the most significant predictor of seniority was qualifications and specifically nurses with one or more qualifications beyond that required for registration were more likely to be promoted into senior and management roles. Findings indicated that male nurses were more likely to hold advanced qualifications and less likely to work part-time, with these two factors accounting for their faster career progress. Family-friendly policies including career breaks, flexible and part-time working were introduced to help nurses remain in their careers whilst also giving time to family responsibilities. These were available to both women and men, but very few men took up the option. It is generally women who take advantage of these arrangements but by doing so, they may be undermining their career prospects. Taking a break from work may lead to a perceived loss of currency that is not easily recoverable. Continuity of service in nursing appears to be positively viewed by employers and a career break, for whatever reason, is a break on career advancement. As Brown and Jones (2004: 20) point out, "family friendly workplaces may not be career-woman friendly". Management in nursing, as in many other professions, is more likely for those who follow a masculine employment pattern (Crompton, 2006).

## Conclusion

In this chapter I have sought to draw out some of the key occupational demarcations in the work of delivering health. Healthcare work is characterised by both occupational boundaries and entrenched stereotypes. As noted above, healthcare professions have a very hierarchically organised power structure and a more complex differentiation than other sectors of the labour force with some of the highest and lowest paid workers (Lindsay, 2008). Across the sector, occupations jostle for influence and boundary maintenance has become an increasingly uncertain process. I have highlighted the dimension of gender both as experience and as analytic tool and have been selective in choosing to principally concentrate discussion on nursing, medicine and management. In some ways, the chapter has been shaped as much by what has been omitted as by the themes included. So, the health work of occupational and physical therapists, mental health workers, pharmacists, dieticians, paramedics, midwives, nutritionists, speech therapists as well as home carers and other support workers has not been considered. Neither, of course, has the important role played by trade unions, professional associations and regulatory bodies in constructing various aspects of the working health environment through the development of policy and lobbying activities – pay, conditions of service, pensions, statutory duties and codes of conduct are all part of the remit of these associated organisations.

The diversity of occupations in the health sector illustrates the multidisciplinary nature of contemporary healthcare. As a result inter-professional working has become more strongly interwoven within service delivery. Another group omitted for consideration is that of the vast numbers of volunteers who give their time and energy to supporting the work of healthcare in various settings – day centres, hospitals and hospices are some examples. There is now a developing literature on the contribution of volunteers to health and this will form part of the discussion in Chapter 8 that looks at different models of care as well as at the divisions between cure and care and the hierarchies associated with them.

Capturing some of the gendered reality of particular occupational pathways has focused as much on men as on women, confirming that the social relations of gender mark out different expectations of women and men and different opportunities that often are informed by traditional gender assumptions. Evidence from the case studies discussed in this chapter indicates that gender inequalities in healthcare work are more damaging to women than they are to men, but this needs to be understood against the wider backdrop of challenges to the status quo – from patient groups, women's health activists and, with the recent greater academic focus within pre-registration nurse training, the gradual emergence of a more pluralistic clinical hierarchy.

The gendered experience of working in particular health professions is illustrative of how gender, though often 'hidden' beneath layers of formal institutional processes, is very influential in the day-to-day work of health professionals as well as being an important factor in individual career progression. Gender has so often been left out of the debate about the status and functioning of healthcare professions, with much space in the literature devoted to the politics of health and the goal of more inter-professional collaboration as well as to the ongoing 'battle' between doctors and nurses for clinical authority (Sheaff, 2005). However, the rise in recent years of a managerialist culture within the NHS has acted as a diversion and, to some extent, has moved the focus of 'battle' to a new arena, with managers and doctors as the chief protagonists. Whilst the power tussle between doctors and managers looks set to continue, the pre-eminent position of doctors in the clinical hierarchy remains uncontested as noted by Timmons and East (2011: 1046) "not only are doctors the most powerful profession within healthcare, and the group with the most status, they are also effectively, the arbiters of status for other professional groups".

Occupational power, clinical status and professional autonomy are pivotal concerns amidst increasingly bureaucratised work environments for health. Alongside expanding bureaucratisation, a greater use of technology of all forms has been another highly significant development in healthcare that has become a technologically-rich work sector (Allen and Pilnick, 2005). Technology changes both the character and meaning of work and whilst technology has transformed both the delivery and experience of health, it is not without its challenges or critics – these are the themes of the next chapter.

# Chapter 6
# Technology and Health

## Introduction

The term *technology* is subject to a variety of meanings depending on the context but Holland (2012: 151) provides a simple but useful definition well suited to the themes of this chapter; she asserts that "technology is all about applying scientific and experiential knowledge to using tools, techniques or systems in order to solve problems or make things easier to do". Drawing on this view, technology is principally about action of different kinds and humans have had a long history of using technology for a variety of purposes. Technologies do not *automatically* work; they have to be brought into use by people and sometimes technology can fail to deliver the intentions of developers and innovators. This means that if we are to understand technologies in healthcare we need to understand socio-technical relations – these are the relationships between technologies of all kinds and the people who use them together with the context in which this interaction occurs. In modern society technologies are often categorised as 'high', 'medium' or 'low' (Holland, 2012) reflecting the extent to which they involve specialised systems or advanced expertise. Over recent decades, the relentless tide of innovation has produced new technologies ranging from bar codes on goods in shops and automated ticket machines to space travel, creating a sense that technological culture seems able to overwhelm other cultural influences.

Historically the links between medicine, health and technology have been well documented with these ordered through wider political and socio-economic forces to construct healthcare as an amalgam of science, craft and technology. In the contemporary Western context, healthcare has become highly technological provided through a range of medical devices ranging from the thermometer to cancer screening tests and from sophisticated surgical interventions to regenerative medicine (Faulkner, 2009). Technology is central to healthcare in advanced industrialised societies and, with its use now so routine, it is rendered almost invisible. Although care work and technical work clearly overlap in health, some are concerned that the rapid pace of technological change in healthcare is altering traditional notions of care work (Lindsay, 2008).

We have come to expect technological medicine with its associated sophisticated heroic life-saving and life-producing tools that extend the normal capacities of the disrupted or ageing body (Schneiderman and Jecker, 2011). Artificial hips, keyhole surgery, blood tests, endoscopes, heart, lung and liver transplants, tissue engineering, genetic screening, artificial ventilation and infusion pumps are seen as standard procedures within medicine that is constantly seeking to break new ground in what is technologically possible in the pursuit of health and the extension and promotion of life (Porter, 1999). Some of the most recent and ambitious technological innovations include state-of-the-art robotics, computer-aided surgery and diagnostics together with 3D imaging – these innovations as a form of emergent technological practice are seen as demonstrations of the boundless progress of technological medicine that traditionally has been a male-dominated domain (Ryle, 2012). Ryle (2012) thus notes the historic link between technology, heroic medicine and male doctors that she claims is linked to status and income-earning capacity.

Due mainly to the enormous advances in medical science and the associated development of new treatments for a whole range of conditions, there has emerged an increased use of martial language and military metaphors within the healthcare lexicon. Such language has long been present in descriptions of approaches to treating disease, but the increased potential of treatments to achieve a cure for a whole range of conditions on a macro scale has led to this type of combative language becoming normalised. Positioning disease as a site of battle, bodies are invaded, we declare war on cancer, disease strikes, we fight insomnia and we bombard errant cells with toxic drugs. Such metaphors bring a masculinist tone to the way in which, in terms of everyday language, we think and talk about illness as a disrupted state of health. The imperative seems to be to counter the aggression of disease with a superior medical force shaped by increasingly complex and sophisticated technologies that may be indifferent to individual suffering and even cause harm. Exposure to radiation through CT scans leading to an increased risk of cancer is one example. Schneiderman and Jecker (2011) associate the imperative to *fight* disease with a moral obligation to rail against acceptance of death, seen by the medical establishment as defeatist.

Medical technology has, in recent times, received increased critical attention in both the health and social science literature, often as part of medicalisation discourses that document how technology has become embedded in the professional organisation and experience of health. The issue of gender and health technology has received only limited coverage and this is often connected to women and reproduction. There is, however, a well-developed wider literature on gender and technology that suggests that technology is a medium of power that is linked to masculinity (Wajcman, 2000) and that there are gender differences in attitudes toward science and technology (Johnson and Simon, 2012). Important connections exist between men's dominance over technology and their power in the workplace. Work settings based on technology help to consolidate relations among men but often exclude women (Cockburn, 1985; Wajcman, 2000).

Against this theoretical background the chapter has several aims. The first of these is through the use of a number of case studies to introduce readers to examples of how technology is increasingly shaping health and health solutions and also the ways in which some of these are impacted by gender. Low, as well as high, technologies are considered, in order to demonstrate how technology in different forms can positively impact health. This is followed by a specific focus on the concept and practice of telehealth (also termed telemedicine or telecare) that is increasingly used to support health delivery in circumstances that make conventional health consultations difficult. The factors of scare resources, geography and dispersed communities inform this section. The discussion then moves to consider the highly contested debate about reproductive technologies which has been the focus of long-standing and often ferocious feminist criticism that sees in these technologies an unmitigated attack on women as discussed in the seminal collection of papers edited by Stanworth (1987). The social dynamics and regulatory regimes that contribute to this controversial area of health are explored with consideration of impacts on both women and men.

A key aspect of feminist critiques of modern reproductive technologies is the manner in which women have been encouraged to defer, with only minimal questioning, to the advances of science. Deferring uncritically to medical science has a wider significance beyond the realm of reproductive health and a number of commentaries now raise questions about the risks and benefits to health and the healthcare system from an unbridled use of a whole range of medical technologies. Scholars such as Faulkner (2009) highlight the social and power relations associated with technology in health drawing out the complex web of interests connected to their promotion and use. Issues of policy-making, regulation, effectiveness, cost and vested industry interests all come into play. A number of different stakeholder constituencies and interactions are involved that make the processes of technological innovation for health contentious and subject to the politics of business and regulation beyond the domain of conventional medicine.

Faulkner (2009) contends that the increased use of health technology is taking place alongside a reduced emphasis on the social management of health with a loss of shared knowledge and practice. This, he argues, has given way to a more strongly articulated individualised notion of health that is culturally driven and state sponsored with encouragement towards 'self-care' as one example. He identifies 'e-health' technology as one mechanism through which individualisation has begun to gain ground, with this exemplifying that the implications of technology use cannot always be predicted. Technology is just one dimension of healthcare but it has come to be seen as integral to a wide range of health interventions designed to restore, transform and extend health and discussion of some technologically-driven health solutions now follows.

## Technology increasingly informing health solutions

The first port of call for those who have concerns about their health is usually the GP. Local surgeries and health centres, as the most common settings for general practice, are not generally perceived to be high-technology work spaces, particularly when compared with many hospitals. Images of patients' paper records contained in labelled buff-coloured folders and stored on shelving close to the surgery reception area remain very vivid for many of us. Whilst the paper storage of records continues in a few GP practices, a majority of patient information is now computerised, with patients legally entitled to see their health records (Pyper et al., 2004). Access to electronic records can support patients in shared decision-making and in managing their own care.

Rapport et al. (2006), reporting on a study that explored how GPs use and reflect on their work space, comment more generally on the impact of computer technology and on how GPs conduct their work. Being able to connect quickly with professional colleagues, as well as efficiently recording patients' care pathways and interventions were identified as two key benefits of computerisation in this area of health. Also being able to readily look up recent information about new drugs as part of treatment decision-making was seen as very useful. However, given the recent emphasis towards more patient-centred care, the computer was seen by some GPs in Rapport et al.'s (2006) study as a mixed blessing, because it disrupted doctor-patient communication. One participant in the study explained this by saying that: "I can't consult and look at the screen at the same time" and another commented that: "the majority of consultations are now computer centred". The same participant elaborated thus: "the new GMS contract has made the computer central to the consultation at the expense sometimes of the patient" (Rapport et al., 2006: 246). Doctors had ambivalent feelings about the increased use and presence of technology in their surgeries, particularly the potential for the depersonalisation of the physician/patient consultation.

Other comments from participants in Rapport et al.'s (2006) study relate to the increasing dependence of GPs on computer technology and their related potential vulnerability when systems crashed. Computer specialists are now needed to join the growing teams of experts involved in healthcare. With consultations nominally restricted to 10 minutes, access to fast and reliable computers was regarded as essential with this making the consultation as much a business as a health encounter. Reorganisation of the desk area to ensure enough space for the computer and printer was another concern with these technologies now very much seen as the tools of the trade. As noted in the previous chapter, GP practices are in fact small businesses and, as such, have to make appropriate provision for the technology required to enable them to operate effectively in both the privacy of the surgery and in the public spaces of the practice. They do this against a background of tightened resources and, in many cases, adapted pre-designed environments.

Much medical success is associated with the development of high-technology medicine that involves the use of sophisticated instruments and equipment developed from modern scientific advances that often have a cross-disciplinary and international base. Enthusiasm for expanded application of these technologies is found amongst both clinicians and those who develop the technologies. Technology suppliers want to sell as much 'kit' as they can to maximise their profits but there can be a disconnect between what the buyers want to buy in terms of delivering health benefits and what the sellers want to sell. Enthusiasm for technology is also found amongst patients who want access to the latest technical innovations and treatments. Some medical technologies have an extended use beyond that originally intended at the design stage. Schneiderman and Jecker (2011) identify the technology of renal dialysis as an example. Originally developed to offer life support to patients with temporary kidney failure, this technology is now more often used to keep patients alive whose kidney failure is permanent.

Technologies of all kinds have over recent years become incorporated into secondary care with levels of technical expertise shaping boundaries between medical specialties. Different forms of medical power are represented through mastery of specific technologies that Serra (2010) argues have come to define particular sets of medical practices. Mastery of a high-tech specialism in medicine confers elite status as well as a significant degree of autonomy. The area of organ transplantation, the subject of Serra's (2010) study, involves a set of hyper-specialised technologies and medical practices across specialisms. Organ transplantation involves the most sophisticated weapons in the technological arsenal, with a spectrum of outcome ranging from at one end, miraculous survival to at the other, death buried within tubes and machinery.

The work of anaesthesiologists and liver specialists (hepatologists) is considered by Serra (2010) to reveal that competency in the use of highly sophisticated equipment is an essential skill in transplant surgery. Opportunities to apply new technologies to surgical practices, was also shown to be an objective of both sets of specialists directed towards the wider goal of constantly evolving new medical and surgical technologies. The push to extend the frontiers of medical solutions through technological innovation demonstrates how the medical division of labour has become demarcated through control of the technical contents of the work, with medical specialists as skilled artisans, wedded to their own particular technologies.

The importance of technology in the form of life-support machinery is nowhere more clearly articulated than in the intensive care unit (ICU) where often life and death hang in the balance. Patients are in these units because they require constant and close attention as well as immediate access to doctors, nurses and technicians who can diagnose and respond to medical crises enacting "technological caring" (Lindsay, 2008). In this setting the use of highly invasive technologies, sometimes as intensive emergency medical care, is not uncommon and patients often cling to life maintained by machines that support and monitor all their vital functions. Hadders (2009) specifically considers the use and withdrawal of mechanical ventilation treatment within an ICU setting in a Norwegian hospital. He contends that it is the advancements in mechanical ventilator technology over the past 50–60 years that makes the ICU possible. He also draws on the ICU case study to argue that death as well as life can be managed through specific technologies.

Schneiderman and Jecker (2011) argue similarly and add that attempts to save life, usually through the application of sophisticated technologies, can be seen as a form of defensive medicine, particularly in the US where medics practise in a highly litigious environment. They further argue that it is at the hands of technology that we have come to expect a seemingly endless supply of miracles from modern medicine. Although it is a mark of our humanity that we shall die, we nevertheless see technology, in the form of machines and tubes, as providing the apparatus to defer our demise for as long as possible. With the development of increasingly sophisticated life-saving technologies, Schneiderman and Jecker (2011: 42) raise concerns about patients and medics becoming "trapped by a dehumanizing technology with no hope of escape". Given that technology for health is a scarce resource, the high cost associated with applying only marginally beneficial technologies is a further concern that carries both ethical and moral implications. Where a patient can be maintained by technology available only in an acute hospital setting, it could be argued that in these circumstances technology has become an agent of qualitative futility, flouting the ethical goal of medicine.

Reproductive technologies aside, there has been very little written about the impact of gender on wider medical technologies, both in their development and application and this is an area ripe for research. Of related interest, however, is the relationship between technology, healthcare work and gender and empirical findings from a US study by Lindsay provide useful insights into the gendered nature of what she terms 'care-tech boundaries' (Lindsay, 2008: 333). Focusing on the work of nurse anaesthetists that has become more technologically intensified, Lindsay (2008) documents how men in these roles being cautious in developing the 'hands-on' caring aspects of the job, were more readily engaged in technological tasks, often with other men. The formation of an "old boys' network" impacted on women who wanted to become more involved in these highly technical areas. These findings are in line with those reported by Simpson (2009) in relation to hospital nurses and discussed in the previous chapter.

The emphasis above has been mainly on the high-technology of medicine that is widely celebrated and now embedded within all Western healthcare systems. Instrumentation developed at the cutting edge of science that has the potential to radically transform people's lives can obscure the relevance of lower simpler technologies for benefiting health and wellbeing. The use of information and communication technologies (ICT) in health is an example of a relatively low technology but one that Balka et al. (2009) argue has a significant gender-technology relation. Through a range of contributions reporting empirical research findings, a focus of analysis by Balka (2009) and colleagues is on understanding how people make use of technologies within everyday life to support health. Within this edited collection it is argued that the internet can add to women's burden of responsibility for locating and managing health information on behalf of others, with this contributing to their role as the *managers* of family health. The editors conclude that, in the context of gender relations, one area that remains under-explored is that of telehealth – the next topic in this chapter.

The role of ICT along with other low-technologies in improving the lives of older women in their nineties is discussed by Loe (2010). Her critique is in the context of women's use of everyday technological tools to help them care for themselves. Loe (2010) argues that maintaining social networks, intellectual growth and community engagement can be accomplished through use of a range of technologies that foster different types of connection. Due largely to differences in age at marriage and women's greater longevity (discussed earlier), greater numbers of older women than older men live alone and, with increased longevity, they can do so for many years. With that in mind, it could be argued that women's ongoing engagement with technology of all kinds can aid independence and enhance quality of life.

Loe's (2010) study, which concentrates on this elderly cohort of women living alone in their own homes develops a type of technological life-course perspective on the ways in which women use and adapt technology to help them accomplish everyday goals of housework, care work, appearance work and health work – work that she characterises as 'doing gender' (West and Zimmerman, 1987). Women used computer and assistive technologies to achieve safety and comfort in their domestic space. Specific techniques included using computers to pay bills and keep track of household finances, maintaining contact with friends and family through email, using reading machines and the use of kitchen technologies to enable them to prepare their own meals. Loe (2010) argues that although communication technologies such as the telephone and the internet may be regarded as low-tech, they can make the difference between life and death and, in that sense, can be socially constructed as a form of health technology. Loe's (2010) argument that, in the face of enormous technological breakthroughs in all areas of health, we can easily lose sight of the capacity of existing technology repertoires to support the autonomy and physical and mental health of older people is powerfully made. Commenting more widely on the benefits of the internet in everyday life, Bakardjieva (2008) emphasises both its social and informational aspects that contribute to the formation of a kind of "virtual togetherness".

Communication technologies have changed the way we live, not just in the West but across all parts of the world. Even in remote corners of Africa, Asia and the Americas, many people have mobile phones or have access to the internet. Global communication technology has been at the centre of increased globalisation that has business, trade and political dimensions. Alongside the economic and fiscal aspects of globalisation, there has developed a globalised market for health that Cartwright (2000) argues has, at least in part, been made possible by the phenomenon known as telemedicine – now more often discussed under the broader term of telehealth.

## Telehealth

Providing scope for the relocation of the site of healthcare, new and advanced technologies have brought sophisticated care processes into patients' homes in ways hardly imaginable just a generation ago. Telehealth, as the wider term to include telemedicine and telecare, links clinicians with each other and/or patients and involves the transfer of information between locations for the purposes of diagnosis and consulting and is used mainly by health professionals (Holland, 2012). The technological possibilities of eliminating physical space and place in healthcare delivery and replacing this with virtual clinical spatial connections have been seen by some as promising increased efficiency and equality in a modernised healthcare system (May and Ellis, 2001). However, the "de-spatialization of healthcare delivery" (Dyb and Halford, 2009: 238) that has the potential to stabilise practice and knowledge over space and physical location, has been difficult to implement and has not been as positively received as some policy-makers had hoped for (Dyb and Halford, 2009).

Telecare technologies, through the mechanism of virtual consultation, enable care at a distance and extend the reach of healthcare to locations beyond clinics and hospitals, mainly to people's homes (Oudshoorn, 2011: 4, 5). Telehealth encompasses services and remote monitoring and scanning devices that moves the burden of care away from hospitals into the community and is a way of reducing emergency hospital admissions. Telehealth systems tend to be commissioned by healthcare service providers from commercial companies specialising in the development of information and data storage and transmission systems (Holland, 2012). Many people with long-term chronic conditions can now have managed care at home. Monitors and sensors are some of the instruments that enable people to screen and check their own health and transmit information to their doctor or consultant via the telephone. Technology enables patients and doctors to obtain real-time data and react quickly to any change in medical conditions.

Advocates of telecare claim that monitoring illness telemedically involves patients more directly in managing their health, though as Oudshoorn (2011) points out, not necessarily taking responsibility for their health. Telehealth also reduces the cost of healthcare to the public purse with an estimated saving to the NHS of £1.2bn over a five year period (Barrow, 2013). Other benefits are emergency services notification for automatic patient alerts and adherence by patients to drug medication regimes. Telehealth is being gradually introduced within the NHS though currently there is some caution on the part of GPs about its effectiveness and sustainability (Barrow, 2013).

One of the advantages of telehealth is that isolated communities who do not have ready access to clinical services such as hospitals and medical centres can be connected to a healthcare provider for information and advice through a telelink. The potential for telehealth to contribute to support in end-of-life care where the terminally ill person is in a rural or remote location is now being acknowledged. Wilson and Mohankumar (2012) cite geographical 'remoteness' as a specific inequity in the potential for quality end-of-life care. Today most deaths are not sudden or unexpected and appropriate terminal care can usually be provided in a planned way. As an example, patients receiving palliative care in some of the more inaccessible areas in Scotland are supported by health professionals through telelink systems and evidence suggests that this has reduced the scale of unplanned visits to hospital (Watts, 2010). A similar system is now being run by NHS Airedale in Yorkshire where the use of video technology in patients' homes enables continuity of care without the need for face-to-face consultations. This process, termed by NHS Airedale as telemedicine, is intended to promote self-care by patients and make them more informed about their condition (Barrow, 2013).

The claim of enhanced self-care through application of telecare technologies is taken up by Oudshoorn (2011) who sees patient self-care as a contested area across traditional and digital care spaces. The term 'self-care' has dual meaning namely caring *for* oneself, and *by* oneself. Oudshoorn (2011) contends that within telecare, responsibility for patient self-care is largely transferred to technological devices greatly reducing care *by* oneself. A further concern is the distinction between technologies that facilitate care and the *act* of care. Oudshoorn (2011) argues that the physical proximity of the face-to-face care encounter characterised by contextualised and personalised communication and psychosocial care through dialogue is not replicated in the digital care exchange that is largely shaped by protocol-driven communication. Oudshoorn (2011: 140) specifically refers to what she sees as the transformed role of telenurses, who she claims are "expected to act primarily as surveillants who control the physical condition of patients based on the information provided by the telemonitoring technology and the electronic triage system".

The gendering of telehealth work is another concern. In the context of Oudshoorn's (2011) research carried out in Germany and the Netherlands, telehealth work arrangements reflect the wider gendered hierarchy across most healthcare professions and organisations. At the telehealth centres visited by Oudshoorn women, in the role of nurses or medical assistants supervised by male managers and physicians, were working at computer terminals wearing phone headsets answering calls from patients. They were trained to follow a set of scripts that pre-structure the work of telecare professionals. Scripts were developed according to the particular technological devices in use by patients with a variety of health conditions and entering data in the telemonitoring database is the first task of telenurses when taking calls from patients. Scripts generate the relevant questions that telenurses should ask patients in order to clarify their concerns and determine next action. By applying standardised categories for action, the telesystems determine how telenurses should respond according to systemically established protocols. During shifts when not answering phone calls, telenurses were expected to watch their computer screens regularly to notice warnings of deviating measures and to phone patients when a warning is signalled (Oudshoorn, 2011: 101).

From the above summary we can see that the invisible work of telehealth workers is highly dependent on a non-human instrument: the phone characterised by Oudshoorn (2011: 99) as an "old media technology". The German centre in Oudshoorn's (2011) study explicitly adopted a gendered recruitment policy, preferring to appoint female nurses to take phone calls from patients because of their social skills and perceived ability to remain calm in crisis situations. These 'phone roles' were attractive to women as an alternative to the physically demanding work of bedside nursing care. They were also generally offered on a part-time basis, enabling women to combine paid work and family care responsibilities more easily, but at the same time, reinforcing the gendered segregation of work in the healthcare sector.

The potential for telemedicine to contribute to a globalised system of healthcare is discussed by Cartwright (2000). Her thesis is that telemedicine has multiple goals: the containment of global health crises, the protection of 'national' health and the enhancement of home care technologies. Hers is a wider vision of telemedicine than most commentators and she argues that "telemedicine is not simply a new approach to delivering health care better it is a method of reordering social life within the framework of global health" (Cartwright, 2000: 348). The exchange of medical expertise and information between places of greater and lesser capabilities can be seen as a move towards a greater democratisation of global health in ways similar to those already operating in national contexts (see Chapter 1). That aside, Cartwright (2000) is accurate in pointing out the non-equivalent dynamic of information flow between settings with very different levels of knowledge – in almost all cases the flow of information is from Western to developing countries. In these conditions the principle of reciprocity on the basis of equality cannot be accomplished.

The case for distance medicine helping to create transnational health identities with blogs and forums pertaining to specific disease conditions is already a reality. New lines of communication forged by telemedicine do, on the one hand, enable remote and dispersed populations to receive expert attention but on the other, restrict this to a technologically mediated form that is devoid of touch and temporal immediacy. The importance of culture to these processes of knowledge transfer in the context of health is considered by Lock (2002) who is clear about both the difficulty and inadvisability of attempts to collapse cultural difference in the name of 'technological progress'. Writing from an anthropological perspective, Lock (2002) reminds us that the successes (justly) claimed by biomedicine that as a discipline is focused on identifying malfunction in the material body, are not free of cultural and moral bias and, as such, may not be readily cross-culturally transferable. The authority of biomedical constructions of health and illness as objective categories has long been contested by social theorists. Dominant and normalised explanations of health often require cross-cultural re-definition and models from other societies can offer instructive (or deconstructive) counterpoints to our own arrangements.

Lock (2002) argues that physical disease and mental distress often have their roots in wider social and political conditions and cannot be understood only as pathological problems located in the body. Interpretation of bodily symptoms in light of medicalised clinical constructions of health may require considerable negotiation in cross-cultural contexts. Although medication can bring relief to symptoms, their underlying causes may remain unresolved with symptoms liable to return. Lock's (2002) work stresses the imperative for global medicine to consider structural factors such as war, exploitation, gender, forced migration and violence alongside the primacy of medical solutions. Medicalisation of health can result in illness being located inside specific bodies as individual sickness, thereby de-politicising its causes. Culture, Lock (2002) contends, is central to individual health worlds and it is culture more than any other factor that shapes understandings of health and illness.

Epidemiologists in accounting for differing rates of morbidity and mortality usually focus on human populations and not on individuals. Because of this, they may have much to contribute to the realm of telehealth in terms of knowledge about dispersed global health communities. Cartwright (2000) characterises this process as a form of actuarial health practice involving the tasks of testing, comparing and questioning all within macro statistical frameworks. These actuarial techniques, she opines, are often used to market telemedicine to particular groups in pursuit of establishing profit-making systems but sold under the guise of a type of *necessary* benevolent paternalism. Because state-based telemedicine often targets dispersed poor rural communities, Cartwright (2000) raises the vexed questions of exploitation (the telemedicine service is not free) versus benefit to the host communities. Alongside, she also explains that the term 'remote' used so frequently in relation to telemedicine has a parallel meaning denoting cultural and social difference.

Whilst the global reach of telemedicine is now well documented, its reception by 'remote' locals has only had limited coverage. In one of the earliest reports on the experience of telemedicine, Allen and Hayes (1994) found that more women than men commented on the dearth of touch and physical contact in the telemedicine encounter though the authors report this finding with caution due to the small response rate. Drawing on views of healthcare workers (in this case, midwives) about a telemedicine project set in a remote community in Norway, Dyb and Halford (2009) found that midwives knowing the pregnant woman beyond the technologically transmitted clinical information made a significant difference to the support they provided during childbirth. Local knowledge of the family context and past deliveries was regarded as important – "what counts as knowledge extends beyond technically derived images" (Dyb and Halford, 2009: 242). Midwives in the study placed high value on sensory knowledge based on smell, touch and sound as well as intuitive knowledge that was difficult to articulate and certainly beyond technological measurement or transmission.

In Oudshoorn's (2011) later study there was a mixed response to telehealth technologies. For some patients (mainly women), the presence of monitoring devices in their homes was an unwelcome intrusion, increasing feelings of anxiety and the sense that their bodies had failed them. Currently a focus by designers of telecare technologies is on the development of devices that patients can use when they are on the move, facilitating the 'mobile' measurement and transmission of biodata from places outside the patient's home (Oudshoorn, 2011). A new generation of mobile gadgets has the potential to improve the quality of life of those who use them but, as commodities in a healthcare market, sensitivity to matters of cost (affordability) and privacy (referring to use in public spaces) may present as challenging to designers and manufacturers of telecare systems. In summary, it seems that there is much to unearth about both the practice and impact of telehealth, particularly in view of its potential as a vital medical service for isolated populations. Discussion of the practice and technology of telehealth has revealed that it is both performative and located, despite claims for its de-spatialising attribute (see above). Although some work has considered the gendered relations of telehealth, this is an under-researched area requiring further critical analysis.

## Reproductive and fertility technologies – it's not just about women

In this section I am focusing on reproductive technologies that are marked by a very specific set of gender relations set within the wider gendered power structures of healthcare. The work of feminist writers such as Michelle Stanworth, Ann Oakley and Hilary Rose (see Stanworth, 1987) has been seminal in this area and provides the broad conceptual framework for the discussion that follows. Some of the ideas considered such as the reproductive subjection of women (Oakley, 1987), may present as 'old' ideas but their relevance for the analysis of the enduring gendered nature of reproductive technologies remains current. Although much of the critique places women centre stage, men are not entirely left out of the frame and increasingly we are seeing commentaries in the health and sociology literature about men's experience of reproductive technologies, often connected to men's involuntary childlessness (Hadley and Hanley, 2011).

An emphasis of early feminist analyses of reproductive technologies and childbirth has been the medicalisation of these processes that has its roots in what Oakley (1986: 136) terms as the "masculinist imperialism of the medical profession". Whilst some might dispute this claim, the history of obstetrics and gynaecological medicine shows that clinical specialist expertise in this area was essentially a competition between male obstetricians and female midwifery (Wajcman, 1991). And it was not so long ago that there was a prohibition against women in medicine, with the BMA still closing its doors to female entrants as late as the latter part of the nineteenth century, along with male doctors openly referring to the biological inferiority of women (Oakley, 1986; Rose, 1987).

Women's reproductive health rights of all kinds have been a central feature of feminist activism for a more female-focused approach within medicine as discussed in Chapter 3. A tendency toward medicalised approaches to childbirth has been enhanced by the routine use of technologies for procedures such as antenatal surveillance and caesarean section as well as the increased technical capability to preserve babies born prematurely. Monitoring for possible pathologies in women's own interests is the explanation given for women and their foetuses being subjected to a systematic medical gaze. New techniques increase choices for women by offering the possibility of curtailing a pregnancy rather than giving birth to a potentially impaired child. Oakley (1986: 138) theorises this watchful approach as the mechanics of patriarchal power and control being replaced with processes of vigilance that she sees as not necessarily improving women's experience and autonomy in childbirth.

Feminists claim that complex technologies focused on physical aspects of reproduction have largely replaced psychological care within reproductive healthcare increasing the social distance between patients and clinicians. The primacy of science in medicine has resulted in an associated drive towards ever more complex technologies that have brought significant changes to the whole arena of reproductive medicine. Although feminist criticisms of technologically-oriented approaches to pregnancy and childbirth continue to be debated, their success in preventing mortality and physical morbidity is also acknowledged (Oakley, 1986). Developments in obstetrics can be life-saving but, while some women are reassured by being surrounded by high-tech medicine, others feel that these procedures, in unfamiliar settings and among strangers, are being foisted on them and are not always necessary. A specific complaint of the feminist lobby is that, instead of standing back and only intervening if needed, doctors are treating all births as potentially problematic and denying women the opportunity to deliver their babies in the manner and place they choose. As a consequence, women are unwitting pioneers on the path of medicalised childbirth.

Feminist visions of health have always directed attention to the social control aspects of medicine and the need for women to assert control over their own bodies and reproductive preferences. Creation of services specifically dedicated to the health needs of women has developed as part of feminist activism and many of these are centred on women's reproductive health that increasingly is the subject of technological advances. Services such as those provided by fertility clinics can be highly lucrative commercial ventures. Discussing the well-documented accounts of these clinics in the US, Rose (1994) highlights that many are not properly regulated and can provide no evidence of success; women, anxious to conceive, attend these clinics and go through treatment programmes that are highly invasive, costly and mostly ineffective. Rose (1994: 186) thus characterises many fertility clinics as "fostering a runaway technology particularly hurtful to women", with this claim still having currency today (Roberts, 2014).

For more than 30 years we have been exposed to the language of reproductive technologies, particularly in relation to infertility, and much of the terminology is now very familiar. Terms like in-vitro fertilisation (IVF), egg donation, donor semen, surrogacy, sperm banks, frozen embryos and genetic engineering have become household terms that some associate with the possibility of historically new concepts of motherhood and fatherhood. When nature denies couples the experience of biological parenthood, medical techniques can offer the possibility of having a child. The associated benefits validate the image of medical and scientific practice as a realm wherein natural obstacles can be overcome in pursuit of the pleasures of parenthood. The work of overcoming obstacles involves patients, healthcare workers and third-party reproducers (egg and sperm donors and surrogates), who with the help of medical techniques, are at the helm of procreative intent (Thompson, 2006).

Whilst the emphasis of many reproductive technologies is generally focused on verified infertility, some techniques such as egg freezing are also seen as a way of alleviating anticipated potential infertility due to the sterilising effects from some cancer treatment as well as through the natural bodily ageing process linked to deferred motherhood (Martin, 2010). However, the manipulation of eggs, sperm and embryos, often outside the human body, gives rise to a number of ethical, social and legal questions concerning such matters as the sanctity of human life and the commercialisation of reproduction for economic gain (Stanworth, 1987). (Traffic in human gametes and embryos, is clearly an issue of social and ethical concern particularly where this operates as commercial trade). Ideologically, children are subjects of social value and seen as investments in the future, but in a collision of values, children in the form of discarded embryos are also the subjects of human waste and this dichotomy contributes to some political discourses that construct abortion as a problem (Furedi, 2014).

During pregnancy techniques to track health risks to mother and baby, including the detection of foetal abnormality, are routinely used in the UK to reduce birth complications; these draw on a range of scientific, engineering and pharmaceutical technologies as part of predictive medicine. Warwick-Booth et al. (2012) highlight a more interventionist approach in the area of maternal health in the UK, compared with some other European countries such as the Netherlands. These interventions, termed by Ettorre and Kingdom (2010: 144) as "the governance of pregnant bodies", are seen by some as an over-medicalised response to pregnancy that is a natural and healthy condition – not an illness. It is not surprising that medics, exploring the sources of foetal health problems, should look first to women as the maternal-foetal relationship is both certain and direct. Unlike paternity, biological maternity is visible and public. However, Daniels (2001) notes that men's relation to foetal health has begun to come under scrutiny as a man's use of drugs or alcohol can profoundly affect the health of children he fathers. She contends that the importance of fathers in creating healthy babies has hitherto been underappreciated and evidence of paternal-foetal harm has largely been couched within a culture of silence.

The 'naturalness' of the reproductive process, particularly childbirth, has become the site of contested debates about the use of technological interventions that are heavily male-dominated. The majority of obstetricians and gynaecologists are male and the increased technological focus of obstetric and gynaecological practice has come under ongoing scrutiny by the feminist lobby. Feminist writers have theorised much progress in this area as the appropriation of women's reproductive capacities by men eager to apply new technologies of various kinds as a way of advancing both medical techniques and their careers (Oakley, 1984). A related and more general point made by Rose (1994) is that masculinist ideologues have been shown to be integral to successfully attracting resources of all kinds for the purposes of research and innovation in medical science. Rose (1994) raises the specific example of the development of gene therapy that, in the US, is led by an elite group of powerful male biologists whom she characterises as being engaged in the pursuit of economic power as well as captivated by the dramatic promise of new possibilities embedded in these forms of innovative and complex technologies.

The politics of reproductive science and technology, termed by Rose (1994: 171) as "reproductive technoscience", is located both materially and conceptually along a continuum of women's rights and women's choices. Controlling fertility through reliable contraception and the right to safe abortion are two issues that have been central to feminist demands for women's reproductive rights and both facilitated by science and technology. Although we have come to see the right to safe abortion as now widely well-established, Ginsburg's (2006: 235) ethnographic account of the ongoing struggle of women in the US to "violate a basic cultural script – the dominant American procreation story – in which pregnancy necessarily results in childbirth and motherhood" reminds us that this right is still subject to challenge and controversy. The opportunity that abortion provides to organise 'disorderly' transitions in women's lives has been subject to political and conceptual manipulation involving the issues of work, nurturance and reproduction as oppositional terms. Principally and as noted in earlier chapters, for women motherhood and paid work are continually placed in conflict.

In some contexts women's choices are determined by powerful *others* as argued by Elson (2004) who explains that in the US working-class women and women of colour are more likely to have hysterectomies, thereby rendering them sterile and incapable of reproducing. Although some feminists have challenged the domain of reproductive technology almost to position this as the enemy of women because of its potential to exploit and control them, the positive benefits to women of technological breakthroughs in aiding the processes of conception and birth have revolutionised many women's reproductive lives (Szewczuk, 2012).

The whole field of reproductive technology is vast and constantly evolving and the opening remarks in this section are intended to convey some of the key 'headline' issues that have particularly exercised feminist thinking on the topic. In recent years a focus has developed on the issue of age-related infertility that has caught the public's attention as more and more women delay the point at which they want to become mothers. More women in higher education and entering the labour market in professional jobs as well as delayed marriage have been seen as major causes of postponed fertility (Warwick-Booth et al., 2012). Hakim's (2006) preference theory (discussed in Chapter 4) is also largely based on the assumption that contraception enables women to construct the fertility and employment balance they prefer at a time of their choosing and without reproductive dilemmas. However, the demands by feminists for women to access higher education, be employed in meaningful paid work outside the home and have control over their reproductive life have brought into sharp relief the conflicting values of production and reproduction that for many women have resulted in unwanted childlessness. Although in the Western world the female reproductive body has become the site of much bio-medical intervention, women have never been at greater risk of unfulfilled desire for fertility.

Szewczuk (2012), in her study of the experience of 22 infertile women, analyses how structuring the use of reproductive technologies such as contraception and IVF around the social practice of postponement sustains the illusion of reproductive control that in reality is leading to involuntary childlessness gradually becoming a normative feature of Western women's reproductive lives. Whilst the value of contraception to shaping life choices for women is strongly acknowledged, the problem it can help to create concerning delayed childbearing has only recently begun to be recognised. Reported success rates of treatment for assisted conception vary but are lowest at around 6 per cent for women over the age of 42 (Szewczuk, 2012). Given the primacy of contraceptive technology in shaping women's fertility choices as reported in Szewczuk's (2012) study, her labelling of IVF as a secondary technology, indicates the extent to which for many women assisted conception is a technology too little, too late.

Discussion of reproductive technologies in feminist literature has focused mainly on the issue of male medical control over the technology and exploitation of women's reproductive capacity. There has been little written about the role of men as reproductive agents in the technologically-enhanced context of reproductive medicine, nor about the emerging new forms of paternity. Technological advances in reproductive medicine that enable the separation of social and biological fatherhood are receiving more attention though associated moral, legal and social concerns have only recently begun to be debated. The marginalised status of men's bodies in traditional reproductive discourses obscures how gender and masculinity are reproduced by the masculine ideal of fatherhood leading Robertson (2007) to comment that infertile men are placed outside masculine hegemonic ideals. The impact on men of their infertility can have profound effects on their views of their masculinity, beliefs about themselves and on their place in society involving feelings of inadequacy, humiliation and fear of being held up for ridicule by peers (Fisher et al., 2010; Throsby and Gill, 2004). A study by Peronace et al. (2007) found that men who had had unsuccessful fertility treatment showed deteriorating mental health, low social support and increased stress resulting directly from their continued infertility. Drawing on an anthropological perspective, Dudgeon and Inhorn's (2003: 45) review of research on male infertility concluded that those who "fail as virile patriarchs are deemed weak and ineffective".

Some recent writing has focused attention on how gendered masculinity has become embodied in sperm and how male identity is challenged when sperm is absent or inadequate to achieve conception. In their research on masculine identities and fatherhood, Dolan and Coe (2011) found that that there was a perceived positive relationship between being male and the ability to father children. One man in their study speaking about imminently becoming a father comments "I suppose it's like a man thing. It's like you feel more of a man in a way … You feel everything's working and you're alright" (Dolan and Coe, 2011: 1023). Identification of masculinity with a potent (and implicitly fertile) male body is evident in participants' narratives in Dolan and Coe's (2011) study that demonstrates how men construct fathering as a highly gendered reproductive practice.

Male reproductive success can be defined as the ability of sperm to penetrate an egg and because penetration is the measure of normalcy, sperm that succeed are deemed as healthy (Daniels, 2001: 317). Characteristics of sperm associated with aspects of personhood confer a type of personal agency to sperm – some documented features are those of heads and tails together with the ability to swim and navigate towards a fertile egg. Defective sperm that cannot accomplish this journey constitute a significant male reproductive hazard and work by Kampf (2013), in the context of male infertility, usefully extends thinking in this area.

In considering the growing intervention of biomedicine to treat male infertility, Kampf (2013) highlights the rise in the importance of sperm in biomedical investigation. In her critique, male infertility, far removed from dominant discourses of men as breadwinners and as fathers, is explored against a backdrop of biomedical technologies aimed at restoring 'normative health' to the reproductive male body. The cultural insistence on heterosexuality is drawn out with implications for 'proper' masculinity that, in the context of male infertility, is presented as a form of vulnerable and broken masculinity. The further concept of the 'healthy body' is also confounded by male infertility specifically because it is *not* reproductive, with fatherhood as the supreme embodiment of masculinity and legitimate manhood (Kampf, 2013: 21).

In terms of reproductive function and dysfunction, the male body has increasingly come under the medical gaze in ways not dissimilar from those most commonly associated with women (Hadley and Hanley, 2011). Focus on the classification and grading of sperm quality along a continuum of healthy/unhealthy suitability for reproductive capacity positions the male body as contested and subject to medicalised investigative techniques that have the potential to undermine male sexuality. Restoration of reproductive capacity to re-establish male virility and mediate the stigma of reduced manhood through compromised fertility is one of a number of goals of contemporary reproductive technological medicine. Male fertility and a range of reproductive practices such as artificial insemination have, in a biomedical age, become socially constructed through the dichotomous paradigms of normality and pathology (Rose, 2010). Gendered norms intersect with cultural discourses to influence reproductive practices that increasingly are being shaped by technologically driven possibilities, particularly in relation to fertility.

## Conclusion

Health technologies are comprised of many distinct fields that are interwoven to create a dynamic picture of change. Scholarly disciplines that seek to interrogate health technologies include sociology, anthropology, history and psychology and this chapter has drawn on these various perspectives to explore both the impact and practice of technological developments in health. An overarching approach has been to consider technologies for health through a feminist interpretative lens. In so doing, I have drawn on a set of sociological meanings to demonstrate that, although there is not masculinist and feminist technology per se, there are values and beliefs within feminist inquiry that question accepted and supposed gender-neutral paradigms underpinning so-called objective, impersonal and value-free science.

Technology is both knowledge and practice and ideas presented in the chapter illustrate that it is the application of technology in health-related contexts that realises functionality and utility to improve the lives of women and men and the working experience of healthcare professionals. Uncritical acceptance of health technologies, however, has been particularly challenged by feminist writers who, though without a wholly unified stance, have nevertheless argued for a more engaged debate about issues of cost, sustainability and accountability. They have also highlighted that technology that is not grounded in social experience is less likely to be useful and durable (Dyb and Halford, 2009); it is also, they argue, more likely to be elitist. The practice of regulation of certain health technologies has only been briefly touched upon above, but it is in this area that feminist campaigners have directed most effort to achieve a more robust and open system of accountability, particularly in respect of reproductive technologies and their impacts on women.

Technologies for health, as well other technologies, are primarily harnessed to the making of money and operate in a culture principally driven by that interest. It is important in any critique of technology and health not to lose sight of this. Technology of all kinds is big business and it is easy to overlook the importance of features such as enterprise and funding in the ordering of regimes for systematic inquiry that lead to technological innovation. Technology also has political dimensions and the priorities for scientific discovery and experiment that are at the root of technological development often speak to projects of domination and manipulation such as war and the production of destructive weaponry. Feminist theory, as one of a number of progressive social forces, has proposed that the contextual values of inclusion and diversity should more strongly influence science and technology as a way of better integrating all aspects of human experience. Sophisticated technologies, as used in health, are complex, dynamic and multi-factorial – that is they are trying to achieve different goals usually within constrained operational frameworks. Feminist ideas argue that technology is not an end in itself but should be harnessed to deliver change for wider social good. An area of health that has seen much technological innovation in recent years through such processes as screening and monitoring is that of illness prevention and detection and it is to the related subject of health promotion that I now turn.

# Chapter 7
# Health Promotion

## Introduction

Health promotion and the prevention of illness have become increasingly central to healthcare provision that is now in Western contexts more focused on chronic and degenerative conditions rather than infectious diseases as the major causes of morbidity and mortality (Kolip, 2010). Avoiding preventable or premature deaths through better nutrition, more physical activity, reduced alcohol and tobacco use and safer sexual practices is the primary goal of the global health promotion movement. The emphasis of the movement is on what causes health rather than what causes disease, with a focus on factors which are protective for health. Protective factors are positioned at both the individual and social level and are developed through education, social infrastructure and public policy. Health promotion, in aiming to enable people to take more control over the determinants of their lives and health, operates alongside protective health measures (such as proper food handling in restaurants) to prevent ill-health (Laverack, 2014).

The range of initiatives and interventions that make up the subject matter of health promotion is very varied and almost open-ended with the term commonly used to refer to different sorts of strategies. Health promotion can be explored through the lens of occupation as in the case, for example, of nutritionists or it can be expressed in activities and processes such as targeted information and health campaigns in the form of immunisation and screening programmes. Health education campaigns are often designed to target individual behaviour; 'stop smoking' and obesity initiatives are two examples that contribute to a focus on what we now commonly term as 'health behaviour' (Armstrong, 2001). An overarching goal of health promotion is to increase awareness of the impacts on health of different aspects of the way we live our lives. Four behaviours in particular have become associated with disease and ill-health: smoking, overuse of alcohol, poor nutrition and low levels of exercise with these behaviours strongly perceived as connected to lifestyle choices (Kolip, 2010). In recent years risky sexual behaviour has also been added to the list of risk factors.

Often, of course, lifestyle is determined as much by external structural factors such as income, transport and housing as it is by personal choices in relation to matters such as how much we exercise or the food we eat. Culture, in its widest sense, is often not only the context but also the working medium of health promotion (the examples of female circumcision and sex education are apposite). In the postmodern world a unitary concept of health is challenged by ideas of culture and diversity making it fragmented and indeterminate.

The ethical and practical framework for health promotion operates along a spectrum of public and private responsibility that is contested due to issues of social difference reflected in both diversity and structural inequality. Given both the complex nature of the overall 'task' of health promotion and the diversity of the population, it is not always clear who should and should not take responsibility for health promotion. The demarcations of health education, public health and preventive medicine, as the three principal domains of health promotion, shape particular interventions that to a greater or lesser extent are distributive of personal and public responsibility. These variously incorporate empowerment and social change approaches that Naidoo and Wills (2009) see as part of a democratic and capacity building model. As an example, immunisation against particular diseases is seen as a public health promotion duty, though individuals exercise personal responsibility in attending to take this up. Health promotion is aimed at local and national populations as well as at specific individuals though Cribb (2002: 263) argues that in contemporary contexts, health promotion is more likely to consist of 'many-to-many' rather than 'one-to-one' relationships.

An underlying characteristic of most health promotion interventions is that they are generally initiated by professionals rather than clients and thus can be perceived as 'interference'. Matters of legitimacy, consultation and power imbalances both between professionals and clients and within communities make this a potentially contested area of policy and practice. Health promotion interventions rely on a range of disciplinary knowledge including epidemiology, biomedicine and social science and are usually presented as social and individual benefit, though the precise nature, extent and value (in both social and fiscal terms) of the benefit are often subject to controversy.

Evaluation of these interventions is thus notoriously difficult and their justification subject to a range of political and social interests. The related ethical questions of how far it is acceptable to pressurise people to change their behaviour in the interests of promoting health speaks to issues of autonomy and empowerment. Dilemmas of individual choice versus public good also come into play and are not dissimilar from ethical conflicts present in the wider health arena. Cribb (2002: 265) characterises this problem as "the individual versus the community", particularly the extent to which the preferences of individuals should be respected if this involves the wider community in paying the price for that individual choice. One way of thinking about resolving the contested issue of individual versus social interest is to consider whether as a society we are better off with or without a particular health promoting intervention. This fits with the founding principles of the NHS aimed at improving the health of the nation.

The above comments set out some of the key characteristics of health promotion as both concept and a diverse set of practices. As noted, the underlying aim of all health promotion initiatives is the advancement of health with this embedded in UK health policy. The delivery of health promotion programmes, however, has not been without its critics. Robertson (2007), for example, notes that surveillance mechanisms are inherent in health promotion and this has contributed to a rise in surveillance medicine culture. The notion of paternalism has also been associated with health promotion with some arguing that inequalities in class, income and education should be more readily incorporated by healthcare workers into lifestyle advice. Sheaff (2005) goes further and argues that specifically citing lifestyle choice as the major factor associated with a higher risk of death is not borne out by the evidence. He suggests that although lifestyle and behaviour are important for health, they are no more important than many other factors and cannot be considered independently of context and circumstance. A further issue is the extent to which individuals and families have real choice or whether this in reality is a choice constrained by limited resources. A disproportionate focus on individual lifestyle and behaviour factors for health is relevant to current debates about the relationship between rights and responsibilities. A distillation of this debate is that there are obligations to take care of our own health and use health services more responsibly but, at the same time, to not lose sight of the social context for health that, as Pavis et al. (2002) usefully remind us, also includes thinking about age and life-course factors.

Another factor influential in shaping health promotion is gender and there is now a significant body of work that attests to the need for gender-specific and gender-sensitive health strategies in recognition of both the biological and social differences of women and men. Women's and men's lives follow different patterns; they have different roles and occupy different power positions in society. That said, as explored in Chapter 2, men and women are by no means homogeneous groups and there is as much to *divide* women from women as there is to *divide* women from men.

The rest of the chapter will thus focus mainly on a number of case studies that each discusses health promotion from a particular gender perspective.

Although, as mentioned in the *Preface*, this book does not concentrate on theoretical ideas in any depth, it is useful to explore some health promotion models that provide theoretical tools for understanding policy and behaviour explored in the various case studies. The next section presents a number of theoretical models that have been used by policy-makers, academics and health professionals in developing health promotion services. This is followed by a brief overview of some of the headline features of what we know in general terms about gender and health promotion. The first of the case studies then follows: this discusses understanding of health promotion from the perspective of gay men with a specific focus on efforts to promote safe sex practices. The second case study takes a critical look at the practice and embodied experience of interventions aimed at breast cancer prevention. Screening for breast cancer is one intervention that is widely taken up but has recently become associated with claims of over-diagnosis and over-treatment of conditions that are not life threatening. The final case study discusses coronary heart disease that in public discourse has been framed as a 'men's disease'. The chapter closes with some concluding summary comments that draw out aspects of gendered health behaviour in relation to illness prevention concentrating on help-seeking and risk.

## Health promotion models – some theoretical context

A number of explanatory models have been developed to aid understanding of the complex web of social, individual and political behaviours that inform the philosophy and work of health promotion. There is a substantial literature on health promotion that has become a separate sub-discipline within health studies. I have been highly selective in drawing on just three models that provide a range of perspectives that I have found particularly helpful in thinking about the topic.

The first model, developed by Becker (1974), is known as 'The Health Belief Model' and is based on the two constructs of threat appraisal and behavioural evaluation. This model proposes that individuals will act to promote their health in four types of circumstance – if they are vulnerable to a condition, if the consequences of the condition are severe, if the recommended actions to deal with the condition are deemed beneficial and if the benefits of taking the recommended action outweigh the costs or barriers. This model focuses on individual behaviour change prompted by careful processing and evaluation of information prior to a decision to act in a particular health promoting way. Becker's (1974) model that is centred on a reasoned action paradigm is helpful in identifying that health promotion is often about competing motivations and intentions.

Beattie's (1991) model of health promotion develops some of Becker's (1974) ideas but presents health promotion as a function of four key elements – health persuasion, legislative action, personal counselling, and community development. These elements operate on a matrix of individual and collective responsibilities shaped by measures that can be imposed by legislation (wearing car seat-belts is one example) or negotiated. Health persuasion is aimed at individuals and is usually led by practitioners. Legislative action limits the behaviour of populations such as in the case of alcohol licensing laws. Personal counselling is usually client-led and individually-based and in most cases will focus on personal development. The last of the four elements is community development that is linked to the empowerment of communities encouraging them to take action for themselves in addressing wider determinants of health. An example of this would be lobbying by a community group to have speed humps installed to slow traffic and reduce the danger to pedestrians. Application of all four elements of the model to a particular health issue may be challenging, but an underpinning precept of Beattie's framework is that if it is applied in a holistic way, a greater range of social, environmental and economic determinants will be addressed resulting in greater health benefits to individuals. Whilst each of the four features in Beattie's (1991) model has its merits, the thrust of much contemporary health promotion appears to focus on empowerment – of individuals and communities, as a driving force in raising health awareness of all kinds.

The third and last model that I want to consider is the typology developed by Naidoo and Wills (2009) that is essentially an 'action model' of health promotion. Theirs is a pragmatic model that identifies five different types of health promotion activity, all of which are represented amongst the case studies that make up the main part of this chapter. The first activity is prevention characterised mainly by the technological medical approaches of screening and vaccination programmes. Largely following the rationale set out by Becker (1974), the second activity is behaviour change, with the need for change generally defined and initiated by practitioners. Education is the third activity and is linked to behaviour change through the provision of advice and information, with choice and control as key aspects. The fourth activity is empowerment that in this model has individual and group features. Developing capacity and skills, though mainly characterised by Naidoo and Wills (2009) as individual attributes, can also apply at the group or community level. The fifth activity draws on the structural paradigm of a social change approach that acknowledges that health depends not only on what goes on inside our bodies, but also on the circumstances and environment in which people live, work and play. Generally the social change approach has in its sights the goal of influencing policy-makers particularly around measures to reduce inequalities. An excessive preoccupation with individual behaviours is detrimental to health when it encourages us, as a society, to neglect the systemic conditions that affect us all (Hubbard and Wald, 1997). A redistributive system of taxation that seeks to transfer wealth from the most advantaged to those who are vulnerable is an example of a social change approach.

The World Health Organisation (WHO, 2005) defines health promotion in terms of processes that enable people to increase control over their health. This way of looking at health promotion is transformational, but it is also simplistic in as much as many of the determinants of health are structural and external to the individual. Acknowledgement of this is an important corrective to approaches that have tended to see health as the inevitable outcome of individual actions and the associated moral judgements about people's personal health behaviours. Risk and risk behaviour, sometimes influenced by external forces, have become integral to exploring different types of health-related behaviours in the contemporary context. In line with Becker's (1974) model, decision-making by individuals to reduce health-damaging behaviour is a function of a conscious weighing up of information to evaluate the potential costs and benefits of their behaviour, but always as part of their social worlds. One example might be the dominant and idealised cultural image of 'thinness' that influences girls and young women to smoke rather than eat, as smoking can suppress appetite (Lips, 2014). The size and shape of the body has come to be a marker of personal order and a cultural metaphor for self-determination. Conversely in this paradigm, being fat or 'oversized' is a marker of being out of control and associated with unhealthy practices and reduced social worth (Zones, 2005).

A common feature of health promotion models is that of a normative prescriptive direction resonating with an underlying paternalistic culture within health promotion as policy and practice. Some (see Naidoo and Wills, 2009 as an example) characterise this as a top-down approach that can be counterproductive. 'Bad' behaviours that *oppose* health such as smoking, eating junk food and not taking exercise can, precisely because they defy normative constructions of health, develop a certain cachet of their own and become imbued with a type of '*street cred*'. Engaging in unhealthy behaviours, though potentially risk-laden, can be the vehicle through which an individual can resist cultural norms – in this case a pre-defined concept of health imposed upon them that may hold limited meaning in the context of their personal lived experience. As Bordo (1993) argues, behaviours that defy dominant social values, as a form of protest, may constitute a symbolic transgression and be highly valued because of this.

Consciously or unconsciously defying prohibitions that are seen to be imposed by remote but powerful others can operate to restore a sense of both individual and group independence from an external moral authority. Rebelling against what we are being 'told to do' can feel psychologically empowering. Psychological dynamics that shape practices of resistance problematise sophisticated as well as overly simplistic health promotion discourses and bring into question related issues of suitability and effectiveness of some policies and campaigns aimed at improving health. The emergence of a more critical health psychology positions health outreach work as a sensitive and potentially fraught domain. Whilst drawing attention to potentially destructive health behaviours, health outreach has also to proactively engage with psychosocial and emotional dynamics, at the individual level and also in relation to social networks that influence choices about health. Bottom-up approaches that more readily engage with the lived reality of people's lives may be more effective but generally only on the basis that issues and choices can be debated rather than being prematurely prohibited.

The challenge to health practitioners is how bottom-up approaches can be accommodated within the more dominant top-down styles characteristic of most health promotion programming. The bottom-up versus top-down tension theoretically directs interventions towards dichotomous systemic positions – not always helpful for optimising intervention outcomes (Laverack, 2014). Intravenous drug use is an example where much health promotion intervention now focuses on safe use and harm reduction rather than harm eradication arising from abstinence – this being an ultimate health ideal but one that is often complex to realise (Campbell and Ettorre, 2011). Fraser (2004) takes the view that health promotion materials enjoining injecting drug users to produce ethical selves through rigid social hygiene-related conduct do need to take account of how individual responsibility and relationships with other drug users can give rise to moral dilemmas and competing interests. Becoming *healthier*, as part of a generally unhealthy lifestyle, may be a more realistic goal of some public health promotion programmes, particularly given the continuing dominance of external determinants connected to social inequality of all kinds.

## Gender and health promotion

Historically most gender-targeted health promotion has tended to focus on women's health needs as a response to women's perceived disadvantage. However, gender differences can also harm men; higher accident rates amongst young men due to their greater risk-taking are one example (Laverack, 2014). Positioning gender issues as the province of women culturally constrains opportunities to develop health promotion aimed at improving men's health. Turner (2004) develops this perspective and draws on claims from male activist groups to suggest that the political importance of feminism might have given rise to an imbalance in investment into research to promote men's health.

Women and men tend to have different attitudes and behaviours linked to health outcomes. For example, women are more likely than men to engage in healthier eating or preventive nutrition by avoiding unhealthy foods thought to be dangerous (Lips, 2014: 149). Where possible, women are also more likely than men to eat the recommended daily five portions of fruit and vegetables. As highlighted in Chapter 3, health behaviours are linked to gender socialisation such that men, as a function of the masculine image of strength and being in control, are much less willing than women to seek professional help regarding health concerns. Ryle (2012: 298) characterises men's reluctance to admit vulnerability and to seek help as dangerous and also as a factor potentially contributing to men's shorter lives. Women, on the other hand, are socialised towards caretaking roles and to be more concerned about their bodies and more readily contact health professionals for health advice.

Health promotion interventions for women have addressed a wide range of issues. Reproductive and sexual health, maternal health, childcare and child development, menopause, breast and ovarian cancer together with osteoporosis have all come under the lens of health promoters (Laverack, 2014). Also, because of feminist activism focused on raising awareness of women's vulnerability to violence from men, campaigns to inform strategies to improve women's safety, particularly in relation to domestic violence, have played an important part in the development of legislation and policing practices to tackle this widespread problem – a problem that, as reported in Jayne Mooney's (2000) seminal study, is 'classless'.

Men's health promotion initiatives have also traditionally focused on a broad range of issues including obesity, drug and alcohol misuse, smoking, prostate disease, stress, sexual health and heart disease. In recent years a stronger focus has emerged in efforts by health promoters to raise awareness of issues relating to young men and suicide (Laverack, 2014). An emphasis of some health programmes for men has been on physical assessment and lifestyle advice, often drawing on stereotypical aspects of masculinity. As an example, the 'Pit Stop' health programme in Australia utilised a racing car analogy to encourage men to engage with its provision

(Courtenay, 2011). Courtenay (2011) cites a growing interest in men's health as a function of a developing men's health movement comprised of a coalition of health professionals, academics and politicians working towards creating a policy environment more receptive to addressing health problems of specific concern to men. This acts as a counterpoint to men's reported lack of interest in their health as a representation of a dominant form of masculine identity that Reed (2013) suggests has been overplayed in medical sociology discourses.

The case studies that now follow have gender as a theme but also incorporate a number of features of the models discussed in section two above drawing out the tension between health as a function of individual lifestyle factors and as ordered through wider structural determinants. The argument made by Woodward (1997) that health and the body are processes of identity related to 'good lives', further informs understandings of the ways in which gender and its reinforcement acts to materially and discursively shape much health promotion.

## Promoting health amongst gay men

Discussion in Chapter 3 of HIV/AIDS briefly touched upon the issue of health promotion in relation to safe sexual practices amongst gay men. In this chapter I undertake a more in-depth critique of the challenges to understanding the health of gay men in terms understood by them as meaningful. This is set against a background of limited information about gay men's health, particularly in respect of how their health might be improved (Adams et al., 2013). In terms of gay men's sexual health individual and social factors come into play as do wider practices of risk and resistance to normative constructions of health. HIV/AIDS infection is no longer fatal and, with the use of a range of anti-retroviral medication, can be well-managed on a daily basis as a long-term chronic condition. Good levels of wellbeing are now being reported amongst many HIV/AIDS sufferers (Liamputtong et al., 2012) who are able to live relatively normal lives though with some level of health uncertainty (Holt and Stephenson, 2006). It also, of course, is not just a 'gay' disease and in many countries HIV/AIDS is spread through the population mainly through unprotected heterosexual sexual activity. Particularly high rates of heterosexual infection have been documented in some African countries. Lips (2014) notes that during heterosexual intercourse, women are at higher physiological risk than men of contracting HIV and that their biological vulnerability is magnified by cultural factors such as exposure to rape and pressure by men to have unprotected sex.

Research by Crossley (2002) is the starting point for considering the role of health promotion initiatives in effectively informing safe sex practices among the male gay community. Findings reported by Crossley (2002) point to ways in which health promotion can be contested and, in some instances, may actually be counter-productive to intended improved health as outlined in the introductory discussion of this chapter. Crossley's (2002) research explored the idea that contemporary health promotion and education can be instrumental in reinforcing risky health practices through its image as 'normative' and something that should be resisted. She took as her case study the topic of gay men's sexual behaviours.

Using a range of qualitative methods, the principal base of Crossley's (2002) research with gay men was the evaluation of a number of services and projects aimed at HIV prevention. Emerging from this work was a picture of gay men routinely practising unsafe sex through unprotected anal intercourse (referred to in gay circles as 'barebacking'), raising the possibility that a huge amount of health education and promotion has had minimal impact in motivating change in the sexual behaviour of gay men. Although the mechanism of self-report as the main source of evidence for this trend does call for caution, there appears to be a shift within gay culture towards 'barebacking' as a legitimate form of self-expression and empowerment. Websites for dedicated 'barebackers', eroticising this practice have sprung up. Notions of intimacy and commitment between gay men, demonstrated through this embodied emotional practice as a way of forging deeper relationships, are articulated by a number of Crossley's (2002) participants. One man explained that:

> the need for the intimacy of actual skin to skin contact is primal ... condoms are not just a question of sensitivity, they are a barrier to physical, emotional and spiritual communion (Crossley, 2002: 56).

Discussion in a focus group with gay men held by Crossley (2002) led to consideration of the way in which 'barebacking', though understood to be risky, was nevertheless experienced as enjoyable, in part it seems because of the risk attached to the behaviour. Risky sex was seen as more valued and more pleasurable and just one of many of life's risks. One participant's comments highlight this:

> I think so much of life in general requires risk behaviour. If you think about it, to succeed in business you have got to be prepared to engage in really quite considerable risk behaviours, so why should we suddenly think that people's personal life should necessarily always be detached from that sort of general way that society operates (Crossley, 2002: 58).

Another of Crossley's (2002: 58) participants posited that some gay men were going "out of their way to seek risky behaviour" and another that this was reactive in that "people become resentful of the fact that they are trying to make everything so safe for everybody". Transgressive acts such as unsafe gay sex are a challenge to the mainstream cultural value of social responsibility dominant within normative health promotion narratives. They also run counter to the rationality that underpins the main features of both Becker's (1974) and Beattie's (1991) models that advocate for health promoters to foster amongst the population reasoned health decision-making on the basis of evidence, education and the wider public good. The social marginal identity and experience of prejudice shared amongst gay men (Robertson, 2007) may explain high levels of risk taking through unsafe sex practices, with gay men feeling that they have very little to lose. This illustrates how a number of discourses are at play within health promotion such that we can see how *positions* are created, resisted and defended both by health promoters and those who are the targets of their surveillance – as characterised by Robertson (2007 – see above).

Other more recent work exploring explanations of gay men's health has been reported by Adams et al. (2013). They argue that although HIV/AIDS remains an important focus for gay men's health, it is not the only focus and that now increasingly the health of gay men, as just one group of men (along with older men and men of minority ethnic origin as two other examples) has become part of a stronger focus on male health in general. Despite this, because gay men view health and sexuality as inextricably linked (Robertson, 2007), Adams et al. (2013) argue that when developing services, health promoters should identify the specific health needs of gay men as otherwise these could be too readily overlooked, particularly in respect of elements that impact sexual health. The specific health needs of gay men include: mental health issues with one in 14 gay men self-harming, sexual health, anxiety over body image, injury from domestic abuse incidents and problems with drug and alcohol misuse (Guasp, 2011). Adams et al. (2013) suggest that gay men's health should be considered in its own right but also that the gay/heterosexual binary that speaks of fixed categories is not always helpful, especially for those with more fluid identifications. This is complex theoretical and empirical terrain not least for health promotion that is more readily suited to supporting more static forms of collective practice and identity.

Gay men's accounts of their experience of health in Adams et al.'s (2013) study develop ideas of wellbeing beyond the emphasis of sexual health. Consulting a dietician and going regularly to the gym were identified as a function of individual responsibility for health, with this as beneficial to all men, not just those in the gay community. Achieving and maintaining good health were seen by the gay male participants as personal responsibility but also as a consequence of external social influences that position 'heterosexual maleness' as a type of benchmark. In New Zealand (the setting of Adam et al.'s 2013 study), gay men could not donate blood and this exclusion was seen as a marking out of gay men as not fully healthy and certainly as not yet wholly accepted in New Zealand society.

An interesting and divergent aspect of the research by Adams and his colleagues (Adams et al., 2013) concerns the perception of some gay men that their health is negatively impacted by images that many members of the gay community present to mainstream society. Negative representations of gay behaviour conveying the dominant impression of over-sexualised and promiscuous gay lifestyles were seen by some participants as contributing to poor health among gay men. The following comment by one man describes this:

> I kind of sort of think we sexualize our culture so much that we, by definition, if you're gay, you must be having lots of sex with lots of men at different times and being completely out there and all over the show, and that's not the truth; well not for me (Adams et al., 2013: 891).

Gay culture that reinforces exclusionary attitudes towards gay men by wider society was thought to significantly set back the important project of the acceptance of gay men. The improvement of gay men's health, particularly their mental health, was associated with this acceptance. The involvement of gay men in lobbying and campaigning activities that, in part, should be directed towards dismantling some of the stereotypes about gay men and gay culture, was seen as essential. The implication of gay communities in perpetuating their negative portrayal was not lost on some of the men contributing to Adams et al.'s (2013) study as one participant comments:

> I think instead of us all running up and down in the Hero Parade (gay pride march) wearing glitter and wearing Lycra shorts, I think it would be more to our benefit to actually model that kind of behaviour, ah, when we are talking about serious issues seriously, a little bit of fun thrown in (Adams et al., 2013: 895).

Jeffery Adams (2013) and his colleagues suggest that the sentiment expressed in the above comment is illustrative of the blame gay men share for their poor health and wellbeing. As called for in Adams et al.'s (2013) research, advancing the health of gay men might helpfully include a stronger focus in public education on issues of diversity and social difference beyond simple labels or categories that can extend thinking on what should be included within health promotion information. A useful outcome from Adams et al.'s (2013) study is recognition that there are negative impacts on gay men's health arising from heterosexism and gay men's minority status that mitigate against individually focused solutions. Health promoting education for family doctors about issues that particularly affect gay men is one example of a structural approach to advocating for health interventions that are more socially grounded. However, as recognised by men in the New Zealand study, this should not detract from wider mainstream interventions aimed at all men such as, for example, the screening for male cancers.

## Breast cancer prevention

Medical surveillance of women and the related use of technology to monitor women's health status within patriarchal medical cultures, have long been of concern to feminists, with this topic explored from a number of perspectives in the previous chapter. For the current discussion, I will focus on some of the controversies related to the use of different medical technologies for breast cancer prevention and begin the discussion with consideration of breast screening. Breast cancer is the most common cancer among women and the leading cause of cancer deaths for them with the incidence of the disease varying dramatically across regions of the world (WHO, 2013). Figures reported by WHO (2013) show that the prevalence of breast cancer is four times higher in Western Europe than in the countries of Africa. Globally a million new cases of breast cancer occur each year (Friedman et al., 2012). Most breast cancer is not hereditary, with only 5–10 percent of breast cancers identified as running in families (Friedman et al., 2012: 3).

Targeted exclusively at women (despite some men being diagnosed with the disease), this health intervention that utilises technologies of medical visualisation together with skilled scrutiny, screens the breast for abnormalities, with the goal of detecting any potential cancer as early as possible. The rationale for screening is that cancers may be identified at an early stage when the prognosis is good and treatment more likely to be successful, thus reducing the risk of dying from the disease.

Screening for breast cancer has a number of elements and includes the following approaches as outlined by Griffiths et al. (2010: 654): breast awareness requiring women to feel their breast for any changes, breast checks by a health professional on a regular basis and mammography visualisation using x-ray techniques that is then interpreted by a clinical expert. In the UK, women in midlife, between the ages of 50 and 70, are invited to attend for a mammogram every three years and are also provided with information about the need to check their breasts regularly as part of ongoing breast awareness campaigns. This is a publically-funded health promotion programme that attracts consistently good levels of take up; the organisation Cancer Research UK (2004) reports that three-quarters of women invited for mammography screening take up the invitation. It is estimated that the programme saves 1400 lives each year. To give this figure statistical context, the Advisory Committee on Breast Cancer Screening (2006) notes that for every cohort of 400 women screened regularly over a 10 year period, one woman fewer will die from breast cancer than would have died without screening. However, public concerns about the reliability of mammography screening have arisen in relation to false negative reports whereby a woman does have breast cancer but this has not been detected by the mammography screening.

The emphasis on prevention through screening has, in some quarters given rise to other concerns related to over-diagnosis and over-treatment, especially for benign breast disease such as calcification common in older women as well as non-life threatening breast cancer. This issue is now a matter of growing international concern, not least because the channelling of funds into screening programmes that are the cornerstone of the cancer industry has not brought us closer to eliminating the causes of breast cancer (Sulik, 2012). However, since mammography screening has become central to promoting breast health, it is difficult to question its utility within a culture that invests so heavily in medical health technologies of all kinds. As Sulik (2012: 189) notes: "screening creates customers, jobs, research agendas, revenues and profits. Those who profit most from screening programs have a vested interest in maintaining the message that early detection through mammography screening is the key". For breast cancer, screening technology has been co-opted as part of survivorship discourses and is inherent in the public character of the disease.

Drawing on feminist thinking, the ideas of Simpson (2000) are useful in helping to unravel the interwoven connection between ideology, technology and the social context in which breast cancer diagnosis takes place. Simpson (2000) identifies three ideologies that she argues shape approaches to breast cancer detection and treatment. The first of these, termed as the technology ideology, draws on pharmacological and technological solutions to problems of health and disease. Development and testing of new drug treatments are often profiled in the media as 'medical breakthroughs' and are indicative of an increasing reliance on science and technology to improve and restore health. This work is also big business and highly profitable for drug companies. The second ideology – of personal responsibility – foregrounds individual factors and is an approach that Simpson (2000) argues is short-term in nature often directing attention away from critical issues such as the environment that have a key role to play in determining health status. The third of the ideologies is the social ideology that fosters long-term approaches and is more concerned with considering communities and social groupings rather than individuals.

These three ideological perspectives draw on elements of both Becker's (1974) and Beattie's (1991) models and point to a pluralistic ideological approach to understanding and assessing breast cancer risk. Simpson (2000) contends that allowing any one of these ideologies to dominate the risk discourse and assessment is likely to result in reducing the number of options for prevention of the disease. In her critique of these three ideological positions, Simpson (2000) discusses the use of the drug Tamoxifen to illustrate the potential difficulty of privileging one of these ideologies over the others. She explores the drug's complex history in terms of effectiveness for treatment and prevention and side effects from its use. Decision-making about its suitability for individual women, she argues, rests mainly with women who are culturally enjoined to do all that they can to avoid getting breast cancer. In some cases, healthy women who are seen as high-risk for the disease take Tamoxifen on the advice of physicians as a preventative agent, but experience troubling side effects, experiencing ill-health as a result. Simpson (2000) argues that the part played by the technology and personal responsibility ideologies in influencing individual women's choices perpetuates a culture of silence about environmental aspects that are damaging to health in general as well as specifically for breast cancer risk.

Health initiatives which promote breast cancer awareness, encourage women to go for screening and de-stigmatise the disease contribute to what Sulik (2012) terms as the *breast cancer movement.* Writing in the context of the US, Sulik (2012: 29) documents how this movement has become highly organised and well resourced and, with increased visibility in the public mind, breast cancer's social status has shifted from disease to epidemic. The development of pink ribbon culture surrounding breast cancer is characterised by a stronger public engagement with the disease and better developed support systems and research programmes. Pink ribbon is now the *official* symbol of breast cancer awareness; the colour pink evokes traditional femininity and the *pinking* of breast cancer has resulted in its permeation by corporatism as a consumer-based culture (Sulik, 2012: 49). Research, fundraising, advocacy and drug development activities have transformed the breast cancer movement into big business, way beyond its beginnings as a health promotion initiative. The core commercial components of this business model are the consumption of medical technologies and the selling of survivorship, with 'survivor' now a separate identity category in many accounts of breast cancer.

Sustaining the breast cancer movement's momentum through reinforcing breast cancer's status as a women's health epidemic is a primary function of pink ribbon culture. Adding a tone of cynicism, Barbara Ehrenreich (2001) opines that collective mobilisation against breast cancer, upholding the image that society is doing something about it and, above all else, keeping the money flowing in, is now the paramount objective of the breast cancer movement.

## Coronary heart disease

There are a number of differences in the pattern of illnesses that afflict, and kill, women and men. One feature of difference is that men experience more life-threatening illness, such as coronary heart disease, at younger ages than women (Lips, 2014). Heart disease is a public health concern in most Western countries and is the leading cause of death for both women and men globally. Heart disease has been framed as a 'men's disease' in health discourses because men die from this disease at younger ages than women (Riska, 2010b: 158). The disease's later onset for women is thought to be connected to the female menstrual cycle. Lips (2014: 144) explains that: "women's oestrogen levels serve a protective function against the build-up of the artery blocking plaque that can produce heart attacks". Thus, because the prototypical heart attack patient has come to be seen as a middle-aged man, physicians may be slow to diagnose a heart attack in younger women, even though women who have a heart attack are actually more likely than men to die (Travis et al., 2010).

Although there is now a substantial clinical literature on the embodied experience of heart disease, there is little published material that explores this condition from either a sociological or gendered perspective. However, recent empirical work by Galdas (2010) that reports men's help-seeking behaviour for cardiac chest pain, considers the impact of cross-cultural factors and highlights men's behavioural responses shaped by culturally inflected variants of hegemonic masculinity. Men from South Asian minority communities in his study did not feel *compelled* to delay seeking medical advice for symptoms of cardiac chest pain. This was in contrast to white men who perceived both disclosing symptoms to others and seeking medical help as a 'last resort' (Galdas, 2010: 226). Galdas (2010) theorises this difference in terms of cultural reverence for medicine as part of responsible masculinity amongst South Asian men. For this group, seeking prompt medical help is male gender-appropriate behaviour. This discussion by Galdas (2010) lends weight to the case for an increased focus on intersectional approaches in the development of health promotion programmes.

Emslie (2005) takes gender as the focus of a literature review of patients' reported experiences of coronary heart disease. She concludes that early qualitative studies were conducted almost exclusively with men and have "tended to generalise from male experience to human experience" (Emslie, 2005: 382). She notes, however, that the literature does point to an increase in studies that include both women and men, though these generally do not have a specific gender focus as part of their analysis. Because of its association with stress, smoking and excessive alcohol consumption, heart disease has thus come to be seen as a male problem and it is men who have been the main targets of health promotion interventions to reduce the risk of heart disease.

This is the starting point of the critique by Emslie and her colleagues (Emslie et al., 2001) that discusses lay understandings of heart disease that they argue renders heart problems in women as 'invisible'. They identify a number of cultural beliefs about the kind of person who experiences heart problems; these centre on those who smoke, eat a high fat diet, take low levels of exercise and who are 'worriers' and more prone to stress. Aspects of physical appearance such as looking flushed or having a red complexion also mark people out as more likely to be candidates for heart disease and, in Emslie et al.'s (2001) study, it was men rather than women who were associated with these indicators. In interviews conducted with 61 respondents, only one participant gave an example of a candidate for coronary heart disease who was a woman.

A preoccupation with masculine behaviours in exploring factors that increase the risk for heart disease shapes public perceptions of the prototypical heart patient as a middle-aged man. Culturally this may divert attention from women who present with heart problems resulting in a slower diagnosis even though women who have a heart attack are more likely than men to die (Lips, 2014: 166). Although the risk for heart disease in women increases after menopause, according to Emslie et al.'s (2001) research, this appears not to be part of lay understandings about heart problems. They opine that one explanation of low levels of awareness is that it is only more recently that the predictors, prevention and diagnosis of heart disease amongst women have begun to be explored in medical research. Healy (1991: 275), writing in an earlier commentary, positions this as a gender issue suggesting that: "the problem is to convince both the lay and the medical sectors that coronary heart disease is also a woman's disease, not just a man's disease in disguise".

Because men have been more readily associated with coronary heart disease, we are now beginning to understand more about male responses to health promotion interventions in this area. One study conducted by Robertson and his colleagues (Robertson et al., 2010) and colleagues explores how masculinities are performed in the context of cardiac rehabilitation. In their research, men recovering from a cardiac episode appear to respond to health promoting activities such as taking part in exercise programmes and adopting a healthier approach to food as a way of helping them to 'get back to normal' (Robertson et al., 2010: 707). These are, of course, two components of preventive strategies to reduce the risk of heart disease. In Robertson et al.'s (2010: 706) research, however, regular engagement with exercise *followed* the traumatic experience of having had a heart attack and assumed a 'vibrant physicality' as demonstration of masculine notions of fitness.

A second type of exercise designed to achieve relaxed physicality and reduce feelings of stress as part of the rehabilitation programme was yoga; this attracted fewer men. Some participants felt that yoga was not for men as the following comment illustrates:

> I think, being a man, men like to do more bodily things if you know what I mean. I think the yoga class would probably be 80 per cent women, the rest men but that's probably men who have difficulty in exercising anyway. I think exercising machines and that are more of a natural progression to a man than yoga (Robertson et al., 2010: 700).

The gendered association of yoga with female exercise regimes acts to culturally restrict men's involvement in this type of activity; non-participation is one way of reinforcing male identity and the sense of a masculine embodied self. A desire by men in Robertson et al.'s (2010) study to be more actively bodily aware in response to cardiac ill-health was still contingent on male appropriate conventions. Men thus were able to retain some element of control over their masculinity despite this having been undermined by a potentially life-threatening health episode. Whilst the sense of manliness might need to be realigned (at least temporarily) in light of changing health, fundamental notions of appropriate maleness do not appear to weaken despite the onset of poor health.

## Conclusion

Theoretical, contextual and empirical discussion of various aspects of health promotion discussed in this chapter, point to health as a personal, social and cultural phenomenon, strongly shaped by gender. Consideration of gender is important for health promotion that has to adopt both proactive and reactive positions in supporting health improvement amongst the male and female population. However, a stereotyped view of gender is as likely to distort policy and practice within health as is the traditional tendency of 'gender blindness'. Thus, whilst a gendered analysis is undeniably helpful, just as important is acknowledgement of the complexities of gender and how roles and identities change over time and how, in turn, these changes impact on health, healthcare and the development of health policy.

A now well established gendered perspective of health is that men are uninterested in their health, with this often influenced by normative notions of masculinity (see Farrimond, 2012 and Thompson et al., 2012 for recent discussion of male resistance to health help-seeking). However, the case study of gay men's health explored in this chapter reminds us of the danger of over-generalisation and of the trap of not interrogating diversity within overarching categories. The relationship between gender and health has specific points of intersection as illustrated by the example of gay men viewing health largely through the lens of sexual health and risk behaviours, especially related to HIV/AIDS.

At its core health promotion is aimed at improving health by encouraging behaviours that reduce the risk of disease and illness. The language of risk is now threaded through much health promotion literature and has informed most of the case studies referred to in this chapter, but risk is not a certain objective construct. An ongoing issue for health promoters is that it is not possible to accurately know all the contextual factors and how they interact to critically determine risk for unique individuals for any given disease. Such uncertainty has led some scholars to talk about the ambiguities of risk consisting of epidemiological findings, causal relationships in understanding how disease develops and the ways in which this translates into clinical practice (see Gifford, 2002). Central to this ambiguity is risk as measured by epidemiologists in relation to a property of a group of people and risk as assessed by clinicians as a specific property of an individual. Translating generalised knowledge to an individual involves the dimension of unmeasured uncertainty and, in part, health promoting activities help to practically mediate risk ambiguity. This is imperfect social and medical science that is heavily reliant on multi-disciplinary approaches to deliver effective and meaningful health outcomes. Given the very wide range of factors that influence health, promoting public health continues to be a challenging and contested area of health service development.

# Chapter 8
# Caring not Curing

## Introduction

In previous chapters discussion of meanings of health and care has drawn attention to aspects that highlight the gendered construction of these concepts as well as to the dominance of the biomedical model of health. This model shapes expectations that ill-health is only a temporary condition that can be remedied. Though public understanding of medicine might acknowledge that some disease processes are complex and thus beyond a 'simple fix', there nevertheless remains a widespread sense that medical science with its seemingly limitless powers will always have something to offer the ill patient. If it *can* be done it *should* be done – this is at the core of the technological and progressive imperative of contemporary medicine that has resulted in medicalisation becoming a key concept of modernity (Bell and Figert, 2010; Schneiderman and Jecker, 2011).

The features of identification, classification, diagnosis, treatment and prognosis together with compliance by the patient with prescribed treatment protocols are the principal elements of the biomedical model, with doctors as its key agents. This medical model of illness breaks down the person into symptoms and parts that are the focus of medical intervention and once an abnormality has become medicalised, it rarely falls out of the clutches of medicine. The scientific base of the medical model is often seen as reductionist and mechanistic, but with a restorative or curative element. It is cure that doctors concentrate on, being concerned with what is 'normal' and what is pathological and making judgements about the boundary between them. And as Fox (2006: 958) poignantly reminds us, it is through the curing of disease that doctors find satisfaction in their work.

The success of biomedicine in tackling disease and illness has been considerable and the biomedical model is now firmly established within healthcare practice, despite critical challenges to its dominance from many quarters (see, for example, Schneiderman and Jecker, 2011). *Acute illness* that often presents suddenly and is short-term in nature is usually successfully treated by biomedicine. Through interventions such as surgery or drug treatment, acute illness can be eliminated to the point where the patient is able to achieve a full recovery. These types of conditions are often referred to in the medical profession as 'acute illness episodes'. Examples of the biomedical approach feature in case studies included in Chapters 3, 5 and 6 and these illustrate in different ways how healthcare is increasingly informed by advances in medical science, technology and drug treatments.

*Chronic illness* differs from acute illness in a number of ways and continues to challenge the limits of modern medicine. The generic term *chronic illness* covers a wide range of conditions and a condition, characterised as chronic, is one for which medical science can offer no cure. Late modern Western societies are burdened with increasing levels of non-life threatening illness and as a consequence medicine is now starting to give greater emphasis to the management of long-term chronic impairment and disability. Rapid advances in medical knowledge over recent decades have brought changes to approaches by doctors in the treatment of some conditions that, formerly regarded as outside the scope of curative treatment, are now considered as chronic. Cancer, once seen as almost certainly fatal, is now for some of its variants more of a chronic illness that can be managed over the long-term enabling the patient to lead a normal life. Prostate cancer is one example. Managing symptoms, particularly the relief of pain, are the goals of medicine in the case of chronic illness. As noted in the previous chapter, HIV/AIDS is an example of a disease that in the Western context has come to be seen as a condition that can be managed, if not eliminated and, as a consequence, has been redefined in medical terms as chronic. Those living with chronic illness use healthcare services but may also be actively focused on practices for self-care as part of their daily routines; insulin dependent diabetics are an example of a patient group that adopts this collaborative approach to looking after their health.

Chronic illness usually unfolds over time and is long-lasting, often with an unpredictable trajectory; it is most prevalent, but not exclusive to, the aged population – those over 65 years (Laverack, 2014). The main chronic diseases in Western industrialised countries include arthritis, heart disease, diabetes, stroke, autoimmune diseases, cancer and oral health problems (WHO, 2013). Some of these chronic diseases can be detected at an early stage of development and can be well managed by drug therapies.

Drawing from the list above it is clear that chronic illness is not a homogeneous category. Despite this, some broadly common patterns of experience apply. Chronic illness can have an uncertain trajectory requiring those with chronic conditions to use different coping strategies to mediate reduced functionality as well as a disrupted sense of personhood (Sidell, 2001). Not knowing what to expect, how quickly the condition will deteriorate and what improvement can realistically be expected from any treatment all contribute to a complex picture of uncertainty and fear.

Tolerating the effects of chronic illness involves holding on to a sense of self, but this can be challenging and come at an embodied cost in trying to maintain a normal life. As argued by Bury (1982), the former sense of a competent self with well established points of reference between body, self and society is disrupted by the onset of chronic illness that for many, can lead to a very changed and restricted life. Changes to social as well as practical aspects of life in the context of chronic illness are discussed by Reeve et al. (2010) who highlight how the biography of self is co-constituted through aspects of both 'doing' and 'connecting'.

Personal relationships are vulnerable to the strains imposed by chronic illness resulting in social isolation for many chronically ill people. Preoccupation with their illness, its treatment, associated embarrassment and a general lack of energy are all factors that impact the lives of the chronically ill (Sidell, 2001). Even where pre-illness social relationships are maintained, these are often subject to renegotiation. Furthermore, the failure of medicine to effectively treat and cure chronic illness *refers* the condition back to the sufferer to be managed by them in the problematic context of the limits of medical knowledge.

Chronic illness can significantly alter the lives of sufferers and can also impact on those who are close to them, particularly those involved in their care. It is the aspect of caring for chronically ill people that is the main focus of this chapter, particularly implications for understanding the relations of care that, as explored in Chapter 4, continue to be subject to gendered assumptions. Care as relational practice and as an instrument of power can be a site of contestation both in formal care settings and in our personal lives.

In exploring how gender is implicated in both the experience of incurable disease and its care, the chapter focuses on two case studies. The first of these is dementia that is now a major global health concern, but particularly so in Western societies. The second is the philosophy and practice of palliative care which has become recognised as a separate medical specialty and one that has gained almost universal social approval (Sinclair, 2007). The social context of death and dying, especially hospice and palliative care, is a major focus of my research and writing and I therefore draw on some of my own research to discuss how this area of healthcare practice is inflected by gender.

## Dementia

A significant aspect of demographic change in Western countries has been reducing death rates and increased longevity in the population with long-term chronic illnesses such as diabetes now starting to dominate the demography (Turner, 2004: 111). The discipline of social gerontology has charted a range of social issues connected to an ageing society, both in positive and negative terms. The literature discussing social aspects of ageing has a tendency to present ageing in both idealistic (successful and productive) and nihilistic (decreasing capacity) ways. Nicholson and Hockley (2011) argue that older people can feel a pressure to define themselves as 'less able' and thus withdraw from existing social interactions that paradoxically can result in increased dependence. Ageing is complex and not just natural or biological. Segal (2013) argues that, whilst we might think that we age by nature, we are insistently aged by culture that in Western societies has an entrenched prejudice against ageing and old age.

A strong influence shaping the negative cultural prescriptions associated with ageing has been the very public growing anxiety of Western governments about the welfare resources needed to deal with the demographic changes caused by the huge rise in human longevity. Segal (2013) points out that over the twentieth century in the countries of the West an extra 30 years was added to average life expectancy, vastly increasing the percentage of people in retirement compared to the numbers of people in paid work. This shift in the balance between the older (retired) population and those of working age has become pronounced in the last 50 years. Of particular concern is the capacity of society to provide care in old age in the context of many people living into very old age with infirmity and frailty, some with high levels of dependency. Many addressing the topic of ageing seem to focus on aspects of cognitive deterioration, particularly dementia, with Downs (2011: 247) arguing that "people fear both living and dying with advanced dementia" and this for very good reason as advanced dementia drastically reduces the quality of life both for the dementia sufferer and their carer. Dementia is often portrayed as a 'living death' for those suffering the disease and a 'living bereavement' for their carers and hooks (2013: 138) comments that "losing one's memory to dementia or Alzheimer's is a way of dying". It is a social as well as a biological disease that, in terms of public discourses and media representations of ageing and 'being old', has assumed a persuasive focus in constructing old age as a time of life to be feared as well as longed for. Miller (2011) takes a particularly gloomy view in his book poignantly entitled *Losing It*, dismissing all possible affirmations of old age and what he sees as the unmitigated disaster that is ageing captured by the materiality of many old people's remorseless decline into second childhood. Segal (2013), however, points out that though the incidence of dementia will accelerate in the oldest old age group, it will still not predominate. This is not the picture often presented in media discourses on ageing.

Although dementia is not a universal experience in the ageing population, it is a condition that has come to be seen as an all too common feature of ageing. The particular challenge of supporting older people with different forms of dementia (Alzheimer's disease being the best known) has come to preoccupy both the healthcare industry and the political class tasked with the seemingly insoluble problem of escalating demand for support for dementia sufferers and their families against a background of scarce resources. Turner (2004) usefully reminds us of the scale of the problem with his claim that Alzheimer's disease is now present in 20 percent of the UK population over the age of 85. In the United States Lips (2014) reports this as a growing problem with 4.7 million people aged 65 and above suffering from Alzheimer's disease. As the population ages, this number is expected to almost triple to 13.8 million by 2050.

A degenerative chronic condition with an uncertain trajectory, dementia affects all aspects of physical and mental functioning though at differing rates. Its early presentation may be characterised by memory loss that is also commonly experienced as forgetfulness as part of the natural ageing process, with this potentially delaying diagnosis of the disorder (see Pratchett, 2011). Cognitive decline is often gradual and can be accompanied by increasing unawareness of people and social surroundings, though this may not occur at parallel rates and in all circumstances (Woods and Pratt, 2005). Dementia reduces and eventually destroys the ability of sufferers to make connections and communicate with the mind – words carry no weight and language has little meaning (hooks, 2013: 138). Downs (2011) focuses on the loss of personhood for those with advanced forms of dementia, particularly the loss of the person they were before the onset of the disease, with this sometimes characterised as 'social death'. A related concern raised by Kontos (2010: 128) is that the loss of personhood can negatively influence the care given to those with advanced dementia leading to their treatment as objects rather than as persons worthy of dignity and respect.

The relation of gender and dementia has not been the subject of many research studies. However, because women on average live longer than men, they are more likely to be diagnosed with some form of dementia. There is also evidence that, in addition to their longer life expectancy, women are at increased risk, relative to men, of being diagnosed with Alzheimer's disease and to suffer a more rapid decline once it develops (Lips, 2014: 180). Besides their greater likelihood of having dementia, women's longer lifespan makes it more likely that they will be involved in caring for a partner, spouse or other family member with the condition (Lips, 2014). Coston and Kimmel (2013) note that in 2010 in the US two-thirds of those caring for dementia sufferers are women and women devote more hours to dementia care than men in similar roles. This care-giving in later life is often understood as an extension of women's care-giving in early and mid-life. Alongside, whilst the ability of women and men to both give and receive care is not contested, the expectations for women and men in these roles are different (see Chapter 4).

Currently more women than men provide or receive dementia care (in part because of their greater longevity) but Coston and Kimmel (2013) argue that if trends continue, in future years many more men (and maybe a majority) will be the givers or recipients of dementia care. Looking at care more widely than just for dementia, Featherstone et al. (2007: 173) report that men are strongly represented in caring for women in older age but also that men as carers have generally been ignored in research. In her research that explored representations of masculinity amongst older widowers, Bennett (2014) found that narratives of caring (for their wives) were significant in constructing an adapted masculinity based mainly on taking action and being responsible.

Returning to the issue of dementia, a question posed by Coston and Kimmel (2013) is whether men give and receive dementia care in ways different from women. By this they mean are men more effective and nurturing care-givers and are they more responsive to the needs of those they care for. These questions are considered in the context of ageing men having to confront a number of challenges related to their self-worth and identity when faced with diminishing masculinity. Traditional definitions of masculinity and femininity powerfully influence notions of how life 'should be' and this can be difficult for later-life experiences, particularly in relation to gender role exchange. Insight into some of these issues is drawn from work reported by Coston and Kimmel (2013). A narrative excerpt from their study richly illustrates this. Ted (aged 77) talks of caring for his wife diagnosed with Alzheimer's disease at age 73.

> What did I know? It was so foreign, like learning another language. I mean, I'm from the generation of men who never changed a diaper for our kids, never cleaned the bathroom, never made the beds. Heck, I can barely fry an egg! But she was losing it – every day, right in front of me, and I had no idea how to care for her. I sort of panicked. I would sometimes go for long drives, so I wouldn't have to be there. I even started drinking a bit. But then I sort of kicked myself in the butt, and said to myself, 'Ted, you got to play the hand you're dealt'. But I won't tell you it hasn't been hard – or that I didn't look at myself, cleaning yet another soiled sheet and think 'What a wimp you are, man' (Coston and Kimmel, 2013: 192–193).

Further narrative from Coston and Kimmel's (2013) study recounts the experience of a 92 year old man diagnosed with Alzheimer's receiving care from his wife. It uncovers a variety of strategies employed by him to mask the disease as a way of preserving masculine sociability as well as him being able to perform everyday chores such as shopping. His wife, so as not to undermine him, had to overlook the purchase of items that she did not want and were not on the shopping list. To remonstrate with him about failures such as these, so simple at an ordinary level, would be to highlight his vulnerability and so contradict the basic tenets of masculinity. This is explained by Coston and Kimmel (2013: 195) thus: "Alzheimer's can be experienced by men as emasculating: the mind's gradual diminishment may be experienced as a loss of manhood". What is also present in this cameo but not explicitly captured by Coston and Kimmel (2013) is the care that is mutually transacted, albeit in very different ways. The cared-for Alzheimer's sufferer trying to help his wife by doing some grocery shopping represents a giving back of care and is an example of how care needs are often multifaceted and set in the context of everyday family life (Bytheway and Johnson, 2008).

The strain on gender identity experienced by men both giving and receiving dementia care may contribute to behaviours of resistance, particularly in the care receiving role. Making excessive demands, asking repetitive questions and generally withdrawing co-operation are behaviours that can be difficult to manage. They also can significantly contribute to care-giver distress (Pinquart and Sorensen, 2003). Although the focus of Coston and Kimmel's (2013) critique is on men giving and receiving care, the problematic behaviours they describe may also apply to women.

Earlier research by Rose and Bruce (1995) discusses the gender implications of caring in the context of dementia and cites evidence to suggest that husbands are less distressed by caring for their demented wives than vice versa. Men in their study report feeling useful with a sense of accomplishment from looking after their wives. They received praise for their caring activities though these were framed by them as feminine or gender-neutral tasks but, never as masculine. Despite the cultural characterisation of their caring tasks as 'women's work', men in Rose and Bruce's (1995) study did not feel that their masculinity was compromised through engagement with care-giving. In the same study women caring for demented husbands focused on the lost relationship with their spouse and did not take pride in the care they were providing. A sense that such care is natural and expected from wives could explain the women's perception of their care-giving as unremarkable and certainly not something for which they should seek or be given approval.

Although the role of care-giver is not an identity but rather a set of practices, care-giving has very much shaped female identity. This is because care unsettles the boundaries between paid and unpaid work (as debated earlier in this volume) as well as demarcations between public and private. Feminist theorising of care has revealed that although care is gendered, it does not mean that only women can care. The entry of men into nursing in greater numbers is an example of how care roles can contribute to masculinity – but not in hegemonic ways. A masculinity of nurturance and care giving is slowly beginning to emerge, particularly amongst younger men, indicative of a growing matrix of variant masculinities (Cornwall and Lindisfarne, 2005). As noted in Chapter 5, though some male nurses move swiftly into management roles, they nevertheless begin their paid caring career at the patient's bedside with this representing a departure from the traditional female nurse stereotype.

## Palliative care

Palliative care is a relatively new healthcare discipline that originated as a response to the inadequate provision of mainstream services for dying people. Now a global movement, palliative care is a recognised speciality that has gradually become more readily incorporated into some areas of clinical practice, despite falling mainly outside the dominant medical model that has cure as its focus, particularly within hospital culture (Kaufman, 2005; O'Connor and Gwyther, 2014). In recent years, however, some commentators have observed that, contrary to its founding philosophy, palliative care has started to adopt aspects of medicalised approaches leading to the suggestion that this area of practice is now a 'guest' of the subculture of medicalised healthcare, because of its growing use of a range of drugs and technological medicine (Watts, 2010).

The concept of palliative care is multi-dimensional and is defined by the WHO (2002) as:

> an approach that improves the quality of life of patients and their families facing the problems associated with life-threatening illness, through the prevention and relief of suffering by means of early identification and impeccable assessment and treatment of pain and other problems, physical, psychosocial and spiritual.

The philosophy of palliative care embraces multi-disciplinarity; affirms life and accepts death as a normal process. It intends neither to hasten nor postpone death and sees the application of palliative care principles as relevant early in the illness trajectory in respect of life-threatening conditions (O'Connor and Gwyther, 2014). Palliative care is, thus, not just concerned with care in the last days or weeks of a person's life, but has relevance at every stage of the disease process from diagnosis onwards (Watts, 2010). In general terms, palliative care can be understood as inter-professional co-ordinated care of the whole person when curative treatment is no longer possible. In this model of care each individual is seen as unique with particular physical, social and spiritual needs, with a capacity to benefit from patient-centred holistic care (Oliviere and Monroe, 2004: 3).

The concept of 'total pain', as a central tenet of palliative care practice, is based on the way in which a dying person's symptoms impact on their physical, emotional, social, spiritual and psychological wellbeing with the goal of palliative care being achievement of the best quality of life for patients and their families within the constraints of a life-limiting illness (Watts, 2010). At the core of palliative care philosophy is holistic care of the dying person contributing to the continually evolving ideology of the 'good death' as a sequel to a life lived to the end (Clark and Seymour, 1999). Because of the highly individual nature of people's lives, the 'good death' is inevitably a pluralistic concept in a heterogeneous world (Sandman, 2005) and in practical terms may be shaped more by notions of a 'least worst death' or a 'good enough death' (Woods, 2007). This being so, a pain-free death seems to accord with most ideals of a 'good death' and effective pain control is seen as a central element of holistic care (Tadel, 2014). However, insofar as this care also extends to patients' family and friends, it may potentially involve ethical dilemmas for the healthcare team with, for example, the interests of patient confidentiality compromised by assumed responsibilities to the family (Randall and Downie, 2006). The balance between making the patient comfortable and keeping the family comfortable may thus come into play. A further point made by Payne (2004) is that not all families are mutually supportive or beneficial to their members. In some cases, family is the site of conflicting interests characterised by abusive, exploitative or threatening relationships.

Although hospices are the main setting and base for specialist palliative care practice, much care undertaken under their guidance now takes place, not in institutional clinical environments, but in the community, often in the homes of dying people (Watts, 2010). Under this model specially trained doctors and nurses give medical and nursing care in a way similar to in-patient hospice services, though usually in collaboration with district nurses and family doctors. Patients with advanced progressive disease are eligible for home care that is provided free of charge (Burbeck et al., 2014). Many general hospitals have established palliative care teams to oversee the end-stage illness of dying patients and provide specialist advice and support to the generalist nursing and medical staff who may have received little training in caring for dying people. Higginson et al. (2002), in their review of palliative care provision in hospital, hospice and home found that one of the most consistent effects of palliative care in all these settings was improved satisfaction for carers and to a lesser extent for patients when compared with conventional or non-hospice services. They also found that there appears to be an advantage of multi-disciplinary over uni-disciplinary teams.

Although end-of-life care has become increasingly professionalised through the development of hospice, there is growing recognition in the literature that the real workforce in end-of-life is usually the family supported by statutory and voluntary services (Larkin and Hegarty, 2011: 197). Currently, much of what we know about family carers at the end-of-life relates to carers of people with cancer though this is gradually changing (Stajduhar, 2011). One of the most significant differences in the experience of family carers is that between those caring in resource-rich and resource-poor countries. In the latter case, the family might be the only source of caring support for the dying person as access to health services may be severely limited.

In considering the social dimensions of family end-of-life care, Kellehear (2012) identifies gender as an important but under-reported issue in the palliative care literature. He argues that because women have traditionally taken responsibility for the bulk of family care and because they are likely to outlive their male partners, these two factors reinforce gender inequality at the end of life. Furthermore as women come to the end of their life, with no-one to look after them and vulnerable to poverty and the lower status accorded females, they are likely to be institutionalised (Kellehear, 1994). Other features of gender in end-of-life care concern care-giver stress, with women reporting higher stress levels from their caring role than men (Goldstein et al., 2004). Kellehear (2012) suggests that men may be more prone to making excessive demands on their carers, so adding to care-giver burden. He makes the further point that because women are culturally *expected* to provide care, they may receive less support than men when caring for a terminally ill spouse.

Whilst Kellehear (2012) has drawn attention to aspects of family-based palliative care, my own research has taken a different focus reporting on the context and experience of care and support given by volunteers to terminally ill people in the setting of the hospice (Watts, 2012). The importance of the volunteer workforce to different aspects of hospice activities is widely acknowledged and Andersson and Ohlen (2005) argue that many hospices could not operate in the way they do without the commitment of volunteers. A recent survey of the involvement of volunteers with direct patient and family contact in the UK as part of specialist palliative care provision found that volunteers are most commonly involved in daycare and bereavement services (Burbeck et al., 2014). Sinclair (2007: 49), commenting on the pronounced voluntary staff component of most hospices, suggests that the population at large sees palliative care and the possibility of hospice support as a gift, and one to be both earned or repaid.

Hospice volunteering is part of the wider tradition of volunteering that is a significant feature of community life in the UK. A core value of volunteering is working for the good of others, expecting nothing in return apart from the emotional satisfaction that such efforts may bring. Stebbins (1996) draws distinctions between types of volunteering: career and casual, formal and informal, and occupational and non-occupational. Gender is also a factor with men and women tending to volunteer for different types of work. Noon and Blyton (2007) argue that women are more likely to undertake voluntary work in schools, with social welfare groups and to engage in fundraising activities; they are also more likely than men to volunteer in health/disability organisations (Howlett, 2009: 13). Men, on the other hand, are disproportionately active in voluntary work involving sports groups and committee work. Fink (2004) draws attention to the relational features of some voluntary work, particularly in the social care field, that she argues can be emotionally demanding, giving rise to emotional distress with the need to develop appropriate coping strategies.

My research conducted in a large well-established English hospice, used qualitative methods to explore a range of topics centred on developing understanding of the experience of becoming and being a hospice volunteer (Watts, 2012). The literature on hospice development has outlined the various ways that volunteers contribute to palliative care services and Hanley (2009), for example, comments on the special talents that volunteers bring to hospice work – painting, meditation, massage, hairdressing and craft skills that can be used for groups as well as with individual patients. With this contextual understanding of hospice volunteering, particular issues for my study included volunteer motivation, previous and current occupational and professional roles, training and support programmes, rewards and benefits of hospice voluntary work and challenges associated with the role.

With the support of the hospice voluntary services manager, a call to participate in the study went out to all of the over 200 volunteers at the hospice. From 17 positive responses, eight participants were recruited to the study with them agreeing to take part in a focus group. Participants ranged in age from 41–77 years and all the participants were women. Discussing this response rate with the voluntary services manager, I was given information about the general profile of the volunteer workforce at the hospice. The vast majority were women and roles seemed to be demarcated along gender lines. Men giving time to volunteer were almost exclusively engaged in more instrumental tasks such as looking after the hospice grounds, driving patients to and from daycare appointments and helping at fundraising events; a few men also volunteered in the coffee shop and as spiritual care workers. Women, on the other hand, were more involved in supporting individual patients in daycare and visiting them at home, running bereavement groups, working on the entrance reception desk, providing complementary therapies such as reflexology to patients, running art therapy sessions and working in the coffee shop used by patients, visitors and hospice staff. The gendering of volunteer roles in this hospice may not be wholly generalisable to other hospices, though Lean and McDermott (2009: 110) note that in relation to volunteer tasks "women are more likely to be involved in direct patient care than are men". Also, the complex and ongoing processes that shape hospice volunteering cannot be fully captured by such a small-scale study. However, the snapshot provided by the data does bring insight to the varied picture of how non-professionalised care is enacted in this setting.

A number of themes emerged from the research, namely motivation to become a hospice volunteer, training and support and challenges of the work that was felt to be increasingly demanding. For the purposes of this chapter, it is the relational aspects of care that will be the focus, with reciprocity acting as an important imperative. The concept of 'giving something back' was very significant in stimulating a regular commitment of time, skills and experience to a number of the hospice's services. Molly, one of the focus group participants, spoke with emotion about her husband's care at the hospice and how she felt she wanted to make sure that others could have access to such high quality care and support. She said:

> he was looked after so well and although it was awful, it somehow made it all bearable and now I feel ready to help out here so that all this fantastic work can go on and others can get help the way we did (Watts, 2012: 109).

Another of the focus group participants, Beryl, commented on what she saw as the real need for more individual care and attention for those coming to daycare, with this explained by Small and Sargeant (2011: 98) as the perceived "gap between what is available and what is needed".

Beryl explained why she enjoyed her voluntary work in daycare but also why sometimes it was upsetting:

> I like it in day care, sitting with the patients and just chatting to them about their week and how they have been getting on. They like coming as it gets them out and they can just be and talk about what's worrying them. You really get to know them … I suppose they almost become friends in a way. Sometimes they can go down hill fast and when they die, it's upsetting and you have lost a friend that you see every week. Sometimes I feel very sad and there have been times when it's taken a lot of getting over.

Eileen, another participant, was aware of the need for volunteers to look after themselves:

> My theory about being a bereavement volunteer is that you have to have lots of empathy and lots of sympathy and love people but you have to have a hard centre. There has to be just that bit in the middle that they don't get through (Watts, 2012: 112).

These comments demonstrate that management of emotions by volunteers is needed to prevent their negative impact and ensure that volunteering at the hospice does not spill over into other areas of life. Whilst stifled grief and bereavement are very much part of hospice work for employed clinical staff, these reactions can be difficult to manage for those without professional training. Compounding the relationship aspects of hospice voluntary work are ethical and value dilemmas as well as the push to be relentlessly cheerful that can add to the stress of the role.

In recognition of these challenges, Dein and Abbas (2005) call for more support and training for volunteers as, otherwise they argue, this work can lead to 'burn-out' as may occur amongst members of the professional hospice workforce. However, unlike professionally trained medics and other clinical staff, who Fox (2006) argues are trained to practise detached concern in order to suppress emotion particularly in respect of death and dying, hospice volunteers are trained *for* concern. Medics and hospice volunteers represent different orientations to death: death does not threaten hospice volunteers' identity as is the case with physicians. Hospice values and cultural norms surrounding death and dying that promote an approach to death as natural, support volunteers having emotional connection with patients as a way of "being an effective companion" (Fox, 2006: 947). This is seen as a specialised task for which training is necessary. A component of the training includes raising awareness in volunteers of the attachment they may develop to patients, but also recognising the potentially negative consequences of becoming too close. Negotiating the balancing act of being close but not too close to patients appears to be part of safe volunteering practice within hospices that, as clinical spaces devoted to care rather than cure as in the case of hospitals, leave room for those who care for dying people to have emotional responses to patients.

Focusing on hospice bereavement services, Osterfield (2009: 139) discusses the potential for 'burn out' amongst hospice volunteers in terms of compassion fatigue, sometimes connected to over-identification with patients and clients. She argues that continually witnessing pain and grief can have a cumulative emotional impact which can sometimes result in difficulties for volunteers in continuing in their role at the hospice. Feeling overwhelmed and insecure in the face of other people's loss is not uncommon amongst volunteers and Osterfield (2009) calls for a greater level of emotional support for them in addition to regular supervision. The task of supervision that Osterfield (2009) describes as helping to move 'head' knowledge into practical 'working' knowledge is not always sufficient on its own to provide the level of supportive care necessary to enable volunteers to function effectively and safely in their role. Confidential counselling and peer support are two approaches that can contribute to developing volunteers' wellbeing and also, as Osterfield (2009: 139) comments, "there is no stigma attached to *resting* from bereavement work for a while". A person-centred approach to care is embedded within palliative care culture and the importance of extending this approach to create volunteer-centric opportunities in hospices within a framework of mutual dependence and enrichment is becoming more widely acknowledged (Howlett, 2009).

## Conclusion

The domains of care and cure are positioned in the health literature as connected but oppositional in terms of the emphasis on relational aspects of these activities. In this chapter I have explored how these concepts have implicit gendered dimensions in relation to professional, community and family care in respect of chronic illness and end-of-life. Feminists have long advocated for approaches that make caring better resourced and more widely shared beyond family ties, but with limited success and this despite growing evidence of more men of all ages assuming greater involvement in care responsibilities. This notwithstanding, because of the increasing recognition of the challenges as well as the benefits connected to the ageing demography in the West, there is an emerging public voice calling for a type of care citizenship model based on stronger user and community involvement in ways mirroring the growth of the modern hospice movement (Small and Sargeant, 2011). Drawing on the notion of interdependence as a civic principle, reducing the isolation of care-giving is central to this project.

Although historically a quick death to infectious disease was more common and certain than is the case today, 'lingering death' from a range of debilitating conditions did feature in earlier times (Walter, 2003). In contemporary Western societies, however, with the eradication of most infectious disease, dying is more often a process that takes a long time and as more disease, once seen as certainly fatal, becomes manageable we are seeing chronic illness as the new boundary between life and death overseen by a variety of professionals. Society's response to this is evolving and is likely to take many twists and turns. Although more men are engaged in care associated with ageing and chronic illness, the language of care connected to loss and letting go, often involving deep grief, is still more usually associated with the world of women and the issue of gender remains centrally located in this debate (Segal, 2013).

# Chapter 9
# Intersectionality

## Introduction

Relations of oppression and structural disadvantage, long the focus of feminist activism, are experienced in the micro-environments in which individuals live out their lives, but these are set within the broader social macro-environment shaped by the politics of all kinds of social difference that inform our identity. The concept of intersectionality recognises that individual identity is multi-faceted and made up of diverse characteristics of 'selfhood', with our gender as only one dimension of who we are and how others see us. Race, class and sexual orientation, as well as gender, are simultaneous processes of identity that operate as institutional and social practice. Intersectionality emphasises that these social categories are inextricably entwined and, as argued by Penner and Saperstein (2013), interrogation of the co-constitution of these axes of stratification has proven difficult to implement within both quantitative and qualitative analyses.

Feminism has been absorbed with theorising difference both between women and men and also, more latterly, between women. As a result, much important work has been done on specific oppressions associated with class, race and sexuality that in its production, has uncovered the critical problems of authenticity and standpoint. This is captured by posing the question 'whose voice is represented here', articulated in Stacey's (1997: 62) claim that: "it is the exclusive prerogative of those who have experienced an oppression or a lifestyle to define its politics". The feminist concept of 'standpoint theory' has thus emerged to be taken up by many in the academy as a way of bringing authentic rigour to their scholarship as well as contributing to epistemologies of the oppressed (see Stanley and Wise, 1993). The adoption of standpoint theory within feminist writing has also been a mechanism for 'celebrating difference' such that attributes, formerly stigmatised, were reclaimed, owned and valued (see, as an example, the work of Skeggs, 1997, for a critique of the intersection of class and gender). Increasingly we are seeing feminist goals engaging with intersecting projects that are aimed at reducing social inequality of all kinds, with this as evidence of Walby's (2011: 151) claim that "feminism rarely acts alone".

As might be expected, feminist analyses of difference draw mainly on the disciplines of sociology and anthropology that offer critical understandings of the nature and cultural production of social difference even within well established hegemonic constructions. Discussion in earlier chapters has drawn on these disciplines to highlight the instability of seemingly fixed social categories. In particular, femaleness and maleness are much more fluid than is often reported and some argue these not to be binaries, but a spectrum of experience and 'being'. A further type of fluidity concerns gender stereotypes that research has shown to vary across social classes (Lips, 2014).

Thus far this volume has concentrated on the experience of health and working for health refracted through the prism of gender relations as one social category. Health and healthcare have been shown to be profoundly shaped by the social construction of gender, with 'what it means to be a woman or a man' as a key influence on experiences of health, even in the face of shifting and reflexive subjectivities. Whilst the social norms of female and male roles continue to inform public narratives about health, families, caring and work, other social positionings are also significant in determining experience of these constructs. If, as I argue throughout earlier chapters, gender is rooted in the social relations of production and reproduction as well as in the socio-cultural and ideological formations in society, how then does gender relate to other social categories such as race and class which are similarly rooted? In other words, how do categories of difference intersect and what does this mean for both individual and collective identity? Further how should other dimensions of social division and difference be *added into* the analysis of individual experience and what people say about their own lives? Whilst it is important to acknowledge that there may be a number of identities at play in a particular context or research project and that this matters, the empirical, theoretical and epistemological challenges involved in this kind of complex social research should also not be underestimated.

Barriers created by race, class, age, disability, sexuality and religion as well as gender contribute to divisive hierarchies that together present us with the theoretical challenge of understanding the impacts of the intersection of these categories on the fabric of individual lives. So often accounts of health are bound up with one particular focus – being a woman, being old, being disabled or being gay are some examples. However, explicitly drawing out other dimensions that highlight multiple characteristics of individual social identity reveals the complexity of interwoven *systems* that, as part of wider social processes and structures, work together to uphold and reinforce cultures of domination. As a result, some individuals and groups are multiply-marginalised. Systems of inequality are intricately entwined and the aim of this chapter is to explore how different dimensions of inequality interact in the lived experience of health and working for health.

The chapter is made up of four parts. To expand the context for the more detailed case studies presented below, the first section considers the tension in social theory between 'categories' and 'inequalities', particularly how inequalities are mutually constituted. The work of Walby et al. (2012) primarily informs this section. There has been a significant florescence of work in the area of intersectional analyses of both health and work, much more than can be adequately discussed in a single chapter. Consequently, it has been necessary to be selective and the third and fourth sections each look at a specific case study of experience. The first of these in section three discusses the intersection of class and gender in contributing to understanding the experience of health. The second case study that is the subject of section four has as its focus the intersection of race and gender in shaping the experience of being employed as a healthcare worker. The chapter closes with a summary of key ideas together with some reflections of my own.

## Making sense of oppressions: theorising 'difference' or inequality?

Feminist analysis has extended its focus on gender as a source of social inequality, to incorporate critiques of the sub-fields of disability, age, ethnicity, sexual orientation and religion and, specifically, the intersection of these that produces multiple inequalities. This has come about through recognition that the prototypical model for feminist theory in its early form was based on the lives of white middle-class women whose experiences as wives, daughters and mothers were distinctly different from those of black women. Indeed as Dill and Kohlman (2011) suggest, it could not be assumed that women from these different backgrounds would even be on the same side of a struggle against racist or patriarchal oppression. They point, for example, to the construct of the family that, though subject to much negative critical commentary from some white women (see, for example, Barrett and McIntosh, 1982), was and remains for many black women a sort of haven and support in the fight against oppression of many types (Dill and Kohlman, 2011).

Theoretical recognition of the importance of intersectionality to make possible meaningful understandings of individual experience has gained greater currency within the academy in recent years, though the approach to conceptualising the relationship between different social groups remains contested. Much of the debate about suitable approaches for the analysis of intersectionality is shaped, not by academic tussles but by political and cultural considerations. As an example, the forced marriage of women within Muslim communities is both a gender and cultural issue but in terms of policies in Western countries, there may be a coalition of feminist and faith interests to address the problem. The same might apply to the practice of female genital mutilation, now seen as an important health concern for some Muslim women, particularly in the West where the practice is subject to legal prohibition. In relation to these two issues a focus only on gender would fail to take account of cultural prescriptions on which affected women draw for their sense of identity and place in the world. In some policy fields, such as health and education, multiple equality strands are represented, with particular issues not reducible to any particular one (Walby et al., 2012).

In social theory and very relevant to this volume is the terminology used to debate intersectionality – 'categories', 'difference', 'social groups' and 'identity' are all terms that feature heavily within intersectional discourses. Of themselves, they can imply a type of homogeneity within classifications but the value of applying intersectional thinking to particular case studies and projects is that it fosters inquiry involving intra-categorical as well as inter-categorical analysis. To illustrate the intra-categorical focus, gender is not a unitary process; rather it is splintered by overlapping layers of inequality resulting in multiple forms of both masculinities and femininities that are internally and externally relational and hierarchical. As an example, the concepts of hegemonic and subordinated masculinities, as discussed in Chapter 2, are indicative of intra-categorical diversity. This, as an academic project, is complex and can lead to the destabilisation of concepts rendering the analysis of substantive matters very difficult (Walby et al., 2012: 231). As a further example, the concept of 'woman' may have a social meaning as an opposing category to 'man', but exploration of the lives of black women, disabled and lesbian women reveals their experience as having little in common with white non-disabled heterosexual women, this leaving the category of 'woman' as not fixed but multidimensional.

Ryle (2012: 55) usefully explains these interlocking identities within overarching categories as a type of *multiple consciousness* that realigns the tendency to see one system of domination or oppression as more significant than another. Gender, class, race and sexual orientation, although distinct social structures, interact dynamically and can be simultaneously experienced by individuals. Zinn and Dill (1996) theorise the way in which these social structures work with and through each other using the conceptual construct they term as 'matrix of domination'. They argue that it is impossible to separate gender from other identities or social categories we occupy. In other words, the term 'woman' is in fact meaningless in sociological thinking without knowing about her class and racial background; some would also argue that the dimensions of age, sexuality and disability are just as significant (see, for example, the work of Thomas, 1999). This demonstrates the potential *emptiness* of categories when considered in isolation. There is no universal experience of gender and gender arrangements are ever evolving subject, as they are, to temporal and cultural frames. Zinn and Dill's (1996) model moves attention from the view that oppressions can be ranked; they also argue that categories of difference within the 'matrix of domination' can produce both oppression and privilege. Furthermore, such is the nature of intersectionality that it is possible to be both oppressed and privileged at the same time.

The 'doing of gender', referred to earlier in this volume, speaks to the way in which we perform gender roles. In the case of multiple features of our identity, Ryle (2012) argues for these to be seen as *accomplishments*. She explains that: "seeing gender, race and class as situated, ongoing accomplishments makes it easier to imagine how they can be 'done' simultaneously. You don't just do your gender in any given interaction; you do your gender, your race, your class and any other identities that are relevant to the situation and subject to accountability" (Ryle, 2012: 56). Intersectional scholarship both challenges theory across disciplinary boundaries and offers approaches to foster greater understanding of multiple complex social relations. For those working in the field of gender equality, intersectional scholarship signals the need for a stronger articulation of other systems of ideological, political, institutional and economic power that impact the lives of women and men as part of the social justice project. It also makes clear how important it is for scholars and policy-makers to resist reductionist impulses in their analysis of issues that cut across social structures of different kinds and of the need to make visible the interlocking structures of inequality.

## Class matters

This section takes its title directly from the important book by the American feminist, bell hooks (2000), written with the aim of bringing social class centre stage in the analysis of structural oppression. The way that we think and talk about social class has changed in recent years, as understandings of class have become shifting and fluid, not least because of the concept of class mobility. This has led some to believe that class does not matter within a democratic society that aims to foster meritocratic ideals.

Traditional concepts of class have largely rested on occupational classification, with manual jobs seen as working class and lower down the 'social' scale than professional occupations (Warwick-Booth et al., 2012). This system of classification, linked to the advent of capitalism, is also concerned with status and power as well as with the level of people's income. As an example, although underground train drivers in London are paid at a level similar to entry-level university lecturers, the social status accorded to these occupations is very different. Occupational identities are often seen as class-based identities. Class is also spatially located but this, too, has been subject to considerable change in recent times with the so-called 'gentrification' of some formerly working-class areas: London's East End is one example, but there are many others. In the reporting of the gradual erosion of working-class culture in these areas, we are reminded that class is also culturally-based.

The intersection of gender and class in relation to health is the focus of Dolan's (2013) recent study that explored how working-class men regard gender differences in health. Men in the study identified a number of factors to account for men's poorer health (than women). Smoking, drinking too much alcohol and poor diet were seen as key issues but they were also mechanisms through which working-class men could have shared status in the context of their every day lives. Women, on the other hand, were perceived to have more self control and so could more readily limit harmful health behaviours. With the maternal instinct, women were seen as having a natural orientation to take greater care of their health and to exercise constraint, particularly in not drinking too much.

Men's drinking featured as an important cultural attribute and was a way for some men to escape the harsh realities of financial hardship; for others it was a reward or compensation for the generally monotonous and unfulfilling nature of their working environment. Hard and often hazardous physical labour associated with working-class male employment was seen as wearing out the male body leading to men dying earlier than women. However, men being prepared to risk their health in this way evidenced their commitment to fulfilling their gender role as breadwinners; it also distinguished them from women and from 'lesser' men, not strong enough to undertake hard manual labour and so live up to their responsibilities. Action, strength and risk-taking were the main features of the masculinised working practices undertaken by men in Dolan's (2013) study.

Men's relationships with their families as reported in the study were principally portrayed in financial terms, emphasising the primacy of their occupations, with male employment as the signifier of men's position as 'good' husbands and fathers. Men's primary ideological position as breadwinners was paramount and this is captured in the comment below:

> You are the provider … the gatherer. The wife tends to the family … I see that as my role. Women like to see a man to be a man … to provide the money … so they have a better life (Dolan, 2013: 8).

This gender role demarcation had perceived benefits for women: from the perspective of these men women were protected from assaults on their health linked to hard industrial work. Women were also not defined in terms of paid work or subject to the same expectations to be engaged in breadwinning employment yielding them a psychological advantage over men. Work-related stress shaped by insecure employment, fear of redundancy and anxieties associated with 'having to find another job' were found to contribute to men's psychological burden, particularly in relation to ensuring that women were not exposed to worrying about men's job situation. One of Dolan's (2013) interviewees explains this thus:

> I get a bit weepy now and again. But if you've been doing something for thirty years and it looks like you're going to lose it I suppose it's only natural … I don't like putting my troubles on to [wife] because she's a worrier by nature … I usually tend to keep things to myself … being a man you're supposed to sort things out for yourself (Dolan, 2013: 11–12).

Men not talking about their worries connected to work or their health was a way of preserving their masculine dignity and a 'strong man' image as well as protecting their families from the often stressful nature of their structural position as working-class men with unemployment and economic hardship often 'just around the corner'. The anxiety about potential joblessness may be accounted for by Ryle's (2012: 373) comment that "not having a job is not just a personal failing on the part of a man, but a failure of his masculinity". Men in Dolan's (2013) study were programmed to work and the prospect of being unable to demonstrate physical toughness through the work of manual labour that signified their worth acted to threaten their psychological wellbeing and damage their self-esteem. Paid work provides men with a gendered identity and a way to demonstrate masculinity; men's sense of who they are is constantly re-affirmed at work which is also often the basis for many friendships. In the context of working-class male culture, Buchbinder (2013) argues that physical prowess necessary for some manual occupations provides potential for men to gain the respect of women and other men and is also the vehicle to acquiring hierarchical masculine status, though often at the cost of their health. Emphasis on physical strength and toughness is a form of compensatory masculinity (Pyke, 1996) that enables working-class men to compensate for their experiences in the working environment where they occupy a subordinated status relative to higher status men who are their bosses and employers. It could, however, be argued that this compensatory model is inherently limited as the labour of working-class men has never been highly valued relative to that performed by men in career and professional jobs.

Whilst men's potential emotional fragility and related impacts on their health were acknowledged by men in Dolan's (2013) study, a more important imperative for them was that of keeping in-tact a valued hegemonic (though culturally subordinated) masculine identity. Male vulnerability that finds emotional expression is not culturally sanctioned within working-class contexts (Connell, 1995; Ryle, 2012); emotion of this type has thus to be kept hidden as, otherwise, this would be interpreted as a sign of weakness. This resonates with the notion that men in socially marginalised positions, such as working-class men, who cannot perform according to patriarchal masculine norms they have been socialised to expect because of the structural limitations imposed by their marginal status, experience a type of deficit that can negatively impact their health. Featherstone et al. (2007) further argue that this deficit can lead to a range of harmful behaviours such as violence or offending and drug use. Risky and damaging practices are rooted in the material reality of men's lives, not simply in their gender. It seems that patriarchy, particularly its underpinning feature of masculine honour characterised by status and regard, may be bad for men's health. However, as George (2014) contends, critical markers of 'honorable masculinity' can have racial as well as class dimensions that are highly culturally situated. And it is the intersection of gender and race that is the focus of the second discussion section below.

## Intersection of race and gender amongst the healthcare workforce

Most of the case studies that have featured thus far in this volume draw on qualitative data analyses to explore experiences of health and healthcare work. In this section, however, I draw on two quantitative studies that each examine the impacts of race and gender for sections of the healthcare workforce. Both studies are characterised by a sophisticated design approach variously involving multiple components and use of linear regression models and statistical controls for dependent and independent variables.

The first of these studies is research undertaken by Karlsen (2012) that reports findings from a project that explored the occupational positions and earnings amongst Norwegian nurses, with a specific focus on gender and ethnic differences. Much research on men in female-dominated work sectors has focused on white men and has tended to overlook the impact of men's ethnic background. More generally there is a dearth of studies that examine intersections between gender and ethnicity connected to occupational roles within healthcare.

Although there is a tendency for men to benefit from their gender (Connell, 2002), not all men benefit equally from patriarchal privilege because of the spectrum of masculinity that ranges from hegemonic to subordinated forms. In white majority societies, white men are generally ascribed higher status than non-white men, have higher incomes and greater access to social networks through which to develop their careers and enhance their social status. Men in female-traditional occupations generally hold the highest positions within these occupations and it is white men who have the most senior posts in male-traditional sectors.

This is the wider empirical context for Karlsen's (2012) study that collected data from a number of Norwegian public educational and employment databases with the aim of examining the career prospects of individuals working in gender atypical occupations, specifically engineering and nursing. The variables of gender and ethnic background, specifically first generation immigrants (those born outside Norway) coming from countries in Asia, Africa, Central and South America and also from Eastern Europe, informed the study design. Findings from the research in relation to nursing revealed a complex set of outcomes and some of the headline features are briefly outlined below.

Management posts in nursing were more likely to be filled by native-born Norwegian men than their female colleagues but, statistically, immigrant nurses (both female and male) had a higher likelihood of obtaining this type of employment in management positions than native-born Norwegians. However, immigrant nurses were most often employed by organisations that provide care for the elderly and the disabled, with this field of healthcare carrying lower status than working in the traditionally more prestigious area of acute hospital healthcare. For native-born Norwegian male nurses there appears to be more opportunity for employment outside their primary occupation. Non-Western immigrant men educated and qualified in nursing are much less likely than native-born Norwegian men with the same type of education to leave professional nursing. The employment patterns of male immigrant nurses are thus more similar to those of native-born Norwegian female nurses than to native-born Norwegian male nurses. Karlsen (2012) comments that this is surprising given that other research (see Chapter 5) has shown that men leave nursing more often than women. A further finding is that the earnings of male immigrant nurses are at least on a par with their Norwegian male nursing colleagues. However, Karlsen (2012) sounds a cautionary note about this finding as it is not clear whether earnings include a measure that accounts for extra hours or overtime payments. If immigrant nurses generally work a higher number of extra hours than their native-born Norwegian counterparts, the results might give a misleading picture of earning differentials. Some further follow-up qualitative interviews with both immigrant and native-born male nurses might have helped to clarify this aspect.

Karlsen's (2012) quantitative study that incorporates a number of variables and comparative foci across the occupations of engineering and nursing provides an intersectional perspective on how gender and race impact nursing employment in Norway. It particularly highlights the importance of taking account of men's ethnic origin when investigating the employment behaviour of men employed in female-dominated occupations. It also lends weight to the value of incorporating a comparative and contextual analysis of inequalities through examination of interaction effects among various intersectional dimensions.

The second case study in this section also has nursing care as its subject. Writing in the US context, Price-Glynn and Rakovski (2012) discuss their intersectional analysis of the impact of gender, race and citizenship in respect of the work experience of nursing assistants who, as non-professionally qualified health workers, undertake the instrumental tasks of toileting, feeding and washing patients characterised as 'reproductive' work. They also perform emotional labour tasks such as talking and listening to clients as well as anticipating their needs. The key workplace features considered were wages, employment benefits (such as health insurance, sick leave, tuition reimbursement and paid holiday) and working conditions with the nature, size and location of the health facility incorporated as a material variable. Drawing on an intersectional model, a telephone survey of 3017 participants was the data collection method used to critically examine relationships and inequalities within and between social groups. Nine-part Likert scales were used by respondents to the survey. The authors cite as an example of their comparative analytic approach how nursing assistant work is experienced by black female citizens versus black female non-citizens and so forth.

Reported findings included a number of inter-categorical and intra-categorical differences. For the current purpose, I draw out the main headline detail to demonstrate both the complexity and utility of intersectional research in this area. Black men and black women fared worst in terms of wages and benefits with white women citizens having the most advantage on both counts. Price-Glynn and Rakovski (2012) argue that for black men there may be stigma attached to the nursing assistant role because care-giving is seen to violate the 'expected' normative culture of black masculinity often associated with violence and being a 'hard man'. Similarly, black women may be negatively impacted by their nursing assistant work that is seen to reproduce and confine them to the archetypal 'mammie' representation.

The components of reproductive and emotional labour were addressed in the survey specifically in relation to the amount of time devoted to each. The nurturing and compassion aspects of care that are central to emotional nursing labour are especially valued. Latina women citizens and non-citizens reported having better emotional labour outcomes than those of white women though they were disadvantaged in terms of workplace benefits. Asian women reported the most time for emotional labour whilst white women and white men, by contrast, reported having less time and institutional support to provide this kind of care. White men citizens report having the least time for emotional labour that Price-Glynn and Rakovski (2012) suggest is due to continued gendered expectations. Asian women, both citizens and non-citizens, report the most time for reproductive labour followed by black male citizens and non-citizens.

White men and women were least likely to work in facilities located in cities where wages and benefits are more generous; this contrasts with Asian women citizens and non-citizens nearly all of whom in the study worked in metropolitan areas. In their analysis of this large-scale data set, Price-Glynn and Rakovski (2012) conclude that race, ethnicity and citizenship categories were more significant than gender. In particular, findings indicated that gendered and raced advantages become more complicated in the analysis when these categories are viewed together with citizenship. They thus argue for recognition of a more complicated relationship between gender, race and citizenship amongst US nursing assistants involving advantages and disadvantages to particular groups rather than a simpler reaffirmation of singular gendered or race-based patterns.

## Conclusion

In theoretical terms the intersecting axes of race, class, sexual orientation, religion and gender are sometimes presented as competing inequalities within intersectional discourses. However, these categories are always situated, contextual and entwined and, therefore, difficult to disentangle in relation to understanding the primary cause of disadvantage. Interlocking identities and mutually reliant systems of oppression act as a corrective to the tendency to see one system of domination as more important or fundamental than another and steer us away from an 'either or' approach to understanding social difference (Ryle, 2012). Gender alone cannot explain individual experience as it is just one of a number of linked processes embedded in discursive practices that construct identity that, viewed through an intersectional perspective, is more fully understood as a multiplicity of identities. Focusing solely on gender to the exclusion of any other type of identity in exploring meanings of health can be both reductive and limiting and, for those working in healthcare, can give rise to health solutions that fail to take account of multiple aspects of marginalisation.

A key feature of the way in which the gender regime has been transformed is the change in focus from the domestic to the public. Specifically an increased presence of women in the public sphere has meant that feminism has gradually been mainstreamed and now is often submerged within intersecting projects. This represents both threat and opportunity – it is a threat to feminism as a separate powerful force for change, but an opportunity for a more connected engagement with other types of action aimed at reducing social inequalities of all kinds. An important message I take from adopting an intersectional analytic approach is that the achievement of substantial social change seems more likely to come about through the formation of alliances across interest groups, each with their own constituency and priorities but ready to accommodate diverse goals as part of the wider social justice project. Whilst I would argue that a more sophisticated and comprehensive analysis of gender will evolve as a result of intersectional approaches, this does, nevertheless, raise questions about the future of feminism that is under threat from a number of hostile forces that position gender equality as of decreasing significance. This forms part of the discussion in the closing chapter that argues for a stronger recognition and articulation of gender as a determinant of health and as a key factor in shaping the experience and careers of healthcare workers.

# Chapter 10
# Conclusions

In this concluding chapter I reflect on what has been achieved through the project that has been the writing of this book together with what I see as the way forward for feminism and gender relations. In looking back across the chapter topics, I draw out some key points that illustrate the significance of gender to the way we socially construct health and healthcare.

At its core this book has been about the quality and subjectivity of individual experience that informs health behaviours and healthcare practices viewed through the prism of gender. Cultural norms and ideologies have been shown to be persuasive mechanisms for shaping understandings of the nature of femininity and masculinity but, as social contexts change, so too do the possibilities for 'being' and 'becoming' a woman or a man. Change served as an underpinning theme of Chapter 2 that set out the principal tenets of the social construction of gender from both an historical and material perspective highlighting how diversity and pluralism now frame gender as both enquiry and practice. The claim that the categories of woman and man are characterised more by intra-categorical difference than they are by 'sameness' is argued for and illustrated in diverse ways throughout the book.

A second important theme that has emerged is that gender is an ongoing process of identity formation rather than a fixed state such that gender is experienced differently within diverse temporal and cultural frames. Gender is something we achieve and perform, but it is also something that can be 'undone' at both the level of ideology and practice. The embodied experience of health discussed in Chapter 3 draws out the ways in which health and illness and expectations connected to help-seeking are rooted in gendered ideologies that continue to influence female and male health behaviours. The power of ideology in creating normative understandings of social institutions was further discussed in Chapter 4 in relation to the family that, despite its numerous forms in contemporary Western society, remains a primary site of mutual care-giving and nurture. Care usually begins in the family and Silva's (1999) theorisation of care as practice rather than disposition that has fostered the traditional gendering of care roles, is important in signifying the possibility for a gendered democratisation of care contributing to a redoing of gender. This, in my view, is essential if women are to continue to progress in the workplace as well as providing financially for themselves and their family in ways formerly more the responsibility of men. The two voices of feminism are those of empowerment and care but there has been an uneven absorption of this double message with insufficient emphasis placed on care-giving as an empowering process for both women and men. I argue that economic provision for the family is a form of care that involves women as well as men leading to the theoretical 'undoing' of the male breadwinner role seen as pivotal to traditional idealised constructions of the family.

Much healthcare work is ordered through demarcation processes that act as mechanisms to protect boundaries across different professional roles in the health sector. These processes have a gendered dimension and discussion in Chapter 5 of nursing, medicine and management critically considered the continuing gendered occupational segregation in health. However, this segregation is not nearly as entrenched as it used to be and we are increasingly seeing gender atypical presence across a number of healthcare professions beyond token status. The extent to which this will impact on gendered vertical segregation in these occupations is unclear though Riska (2010a) argues that in the case of medicine gender stereotyping, discrimination in medical schools and inflexible work patterns, place women at a disadvantage resulting in the lack of advancement of female doctors into leadership positions in academic medicine and in the high status specialties.

Optimism about opportunities for women to take up senior posts in the wider healthcare sector in significant numbers, even if not on a par with men, remains muted due to the persistence in healthcare organisations of embedded gendered values and structures. Although we have seen a shift in the nature of gender relations, we should not overlook the way in which male hegemony and an unreconstructed masculine view of the world prevail in the upper echelons of healthcare. More men than women derive power and status from health systems as they are currently configured and therefore have an interest in defending the status quo. Paradoxically, this does not appear to be benefiting men's health in terms of life expectancy given that this is approximately four years less for men than it is for women (Roberstson, 2007). Explanations for this paradox comprise a combination of factors including higher rates of death by accident and suicide amongst younger men, greater levels of obesity in men of all ages and their greater consumption of alcohol together with higher levels of illicit drug-taking amongst the male population (Robertson, 2007).

The significance of technology in changing all areas of health and healthcare was the subject of Chapter 6. Discussion highlighted how increasingly health has become a technologically rich sector with low and high level technologies providing a range of possibilities for improving health, extending life and ameliorating harmful side effects of harsh medical treatments. Science and technology have triumphed within healthcare, particularly medicine. Much writing on this topic draws on the assumption that technologies for health are gender neutral in the sense that they are aimed at a universal advancement of health. However, feminist critiques of the use and development of health technologies point to the ways in which issues of access, cost, sustainability, corporate priorities and accountability are often overlooked in discussion of the benefits derived from their application. Telecare, as an emerging health practice that is heavily technology dependent, also featured in the chapter. This new way of delivering health services has the potential to change the way we access healthcare and not just amongst remote communities. However, Oudshoorn's (2011) critique of the development of telecare is a powerful reminder that all technological systems require workers to operate and monitor them and that these systems are never fully automated. In the organisations that featured in Oudshoorn's (2011) research, it was almost entirely women who were found to be working on the front line of telecare in low status call centre operator roles, reinforcing the gendered segregation of work within the healthcare sector.

The technological theme was continued in Chapter 7 that discussed a number of health promotion theories and strategies. Practices of screening and testing are important within health promotion that increasingly is focused on measures to improve health and prevent illness. Gender is recognised as a prominent dimension of health promotion and the selected case studies explored the ways in which learned gender roles impact on lifestyle choices and health behaviours. However, diverse experiences of femininity and masculinity discussed in the chapter indicate that health promotion approaches focusing on simplistic and stereotyped meanings of gender may be counter-productive to the goal of effective education about health. Progress towards health improvement and greater health equality rests on policy-makers and health practitioners working with new and diverse patterns of attitude and behaviour. Top-down instruction is giving way to dialogue and reciprocal learning, with the infallibility of medical science now widely challenged, not least due to widespread use of the internet and greater accessibility of information on health-related topics. Debates about health and medical knowledge are no longer restricted to medical circles and trust in medics is on the decline (Nettleton and Gustafsson, 2002: 6). Increasingly individuals are deciding for themselves about choices for health and participating in their own healthcare on their own terms; gender roles shaped by cultural norms continue to strongly influence those choices.

Reference to the dominance of the biomedical model of health, with its focus on the curing of disease, recurs throughout this volume, so the emphasis of Chapter 8 on care rather than cure, feels like an 'off course' deviation, but one that I considered important to make. Despite the huge advances in medical science over the past century, not all disease can be cured. The high-tech culture of medicine that sees death as failure makes acknowledgement of the reality that, whilst some conditions though treatable in the short term, are in the longer term incurable, at best very difficult. The availability of new drug therapies, better diagnostic instrumentation and innovative surgical techniques all contribute to an image of disease as something that can be 'beaten'. The chapter's case studies of dementia and palliative care, however, demonstrate the importance of care when cure is not possible; they also interrogate how the gendering of care at the end of life reflects wider social roles and gendered patterns of health. Whilst the case study of dementia care illustrates how gender can fluctuate in nature and intensity in response to life-course challenges, the discussion of palliative care in the context of hospice volunteering suggests that the work of emotional caring labour is more readily taken up by women, with this seen as an extension of women's caring role in the family.

Health and working for health have been shown to be constructed through a number of social processes and, whilst gender has been central to the analysis presented in this book, other social differences need to be factored in when tackling the challenging task of understanding the sources of health inequalities. The topic of intersectionality is, therefore, important in helping to avoid the dangers of generalisation and oversimplification whereby the differences among women and men are overlooked. The potential for health improvement strategies to entrench gender stereotyping is another concern (one example being the early HIV/AIDS campaigns that underscored the message that HIV/AIDS is primarily a 'gay' disease). These points and the case studies presented in Chapter 9 illustrate why we need a complex understanding not only of the multiple determinants of health and the multiple components of gender identity, but also of the interaction between gender and other factors such as race, class, sexuality, age and disability.

These considerations apply equally to healthcare practice. The attitudes of clinicians and the quality of their relationships with health service users are influenced by age, gender and ethnicity because their professional behaviour inevitably draws on their own personal life experience as well as their training. Their approaches to patients can, in turn, elicit a more or less positive response from patients, making their health interventions more or less effective. Research reported by Hippisley-Cox et al. (2000) found that general practices employing female doctors, younger doctors or more practice nurses had lower rates of teenage pregnancy. Social divisions of all kinds are reflected in both the delivery and use of health services and, whilst feminist activism has been highly successful in raising awareness of gender as significant for health, commentators are increasingly arguing that cultural and socio-economic factors are of parallel importance to understanding the causes of health inequality.

## The future of gender and feminism

Health and healthcare are profoundly affected by sex and gender differences and there are few aspects of health or of healthcare systems in Western societies that are not experienced differently by women and men or shaped by the biological or social differences between them. Right across the health spectrum, from personal behaviour, morbidity and mortality rates through to patterns of demand for services and employment in health-related professions and occupations, there are significant differences in the ways in which women and men experience health and healthcare. Although we now have a deeper grasp of the social construction of both gender and health and their related impacts on health outcomes for individuals and families, gender has, until relatively recently, been overlooked or uncontested and kept on the margins of public policy and political debate.

The change to this position, with the relationship between gender and health being made explicit within mainstream sociological and policy discourses, really took hold in the 1970s when feminists began to challenge medical orthodoxies that historically had constructed health as a matter of biology and gender as an entirely natural phenomenon. Feminists challenging patriarchal systems and campaigning for women to have control over their bodies, to participate in healthcare on their own terms that sometimes involved exposing the fallibility of the medical establishment and bringing centre stage the value of women's experiential knowledge, resulted in the emergence of a new gender politics of health. This was intrinsically controversial because of feminism's contestation of established institutions and power structures and also because of its growing influence that led to feminist projects building their own institutions (Walby, 2011). Despite critical and 'backlash' responses (led mainly but not exclusively by men) that include misrepresentation, attempts to re-domesticate women and ridiculing of feminist demands by the media, feminist gains have been considerable (Faludi, 1991; Walby, 2011). The right to effective birth control, safe abortion and more female-friendly healthcare and maternity services are some of the material accomplishments of feminism.

The links made by feminist researchers between women's ill-health and the unequal distribution of power and opportunity between women and men in patriarchal systems continue to call attention to the need for a focus on the specific health needs of women. As a result, there have been great gains for women and the establishment of a global women's health movement now formally incorporated into the work of the World Health Organisation might suggest that feminism's work, as far as women's health is concerned, is more or less done. However, the account in this volume of the strength of feminism is not an argument that all feminist goals have been achieved and discussion herein demonstrates the ongoing and continually evolving project of feminism and the remaining challenges it faces in the context of persistent structural and systemic inequality.

The feminist movement, whilst advancing women's interests, has also through its contribution to the development of a substantial body of writing on gender that includes the theorisation of masculinities, directed attention to issues that impact on men as a diverse category. By contesting the conventional definition of masculinity, feminism created a theoretical and experiential 'space' for men to start to question it too. As Connell (2002: 79) explains: "because gender practice involves bodies but is not biologically determined, the gender practice being learned may actually be hostile to bodies' physical well-being". The reluctance of men to seek help for illness because it is unmanly to admit pain and appear weak illustrates Connell's (2002) point. Feminist backlash discourses which claim that feminism has overstepped the equality boundary in making ever more vociferous demands for women's rights at the expense of those of men (Faludi, 1991) fail to recognise the role of feminism in giving voice to issues that impact men. The case of men's health, that until relatively recently has failed to be seen in policy terms as a separate serious concern, this despite the evidence of men's poorer rates of morbidity and mortality, is a good example. This issue would not have got onto the health agenda if feminists had not placed gender on the policy map.

In its earliest form feminism was understandably focused on action to bring about change in female consciousness as a precondition for achieving material improvements in women's lives. Feminist projects across many domains such as the economy, the workplace, the home and in the arts were engaged with imagining the transformation of gender relations and these using a variety of approaches ranging from large-scale marches and demonstrations to literary campaigns – there is no single way 'to do' feminism. In the modern age feminism is being increasingly defined by technology with tools that enable women and men to build a strong and reactive movement online and across virtual spaces. Despite increased opportunities for cross-national and intersecting feminist projects, there are new and growing political, environmental and financial crises threatening feminism and these should not be underestimated in terms of their potential to claw back some of the gains secured for women from feminist activism (Walby, 2011).

Feminism continues in new and plural forms and the movement's concerns are forever shifting, embracing new coalitions and networks forging alliances at the local, national and global level leading to the expansion of the feminist project. Indeed and as pointed out by Connell (2002), there are significant aspects of gender relations that cannot be understood locally and that require analysis on a global scale. Discussion in the previous chapter demonstrated that such analyses increasingly involve the incorporation of feminist perspectives alongside other equality objectives and, within feminism, a commitment to ensuring that differences between women are adequately addressed. The intersection of gender inequality with other inequalities is undoubtedly a challenge for feminism. One possible consequence is that in the future feminism may be less visible as a separately identified form of organisation giving rise to the impression that feminism has become diluted or has even faded away. This carries potential implications for the future analysis of the contribution of feminism to social change and illustrates the theoretical and practical tensions associated with maintaining gender as an important analytical focus within intersecting projects. Nevertheless, if feminism as a movement is well allied, as seems to be emerging, then the outlook for its continuing effectiveness as a significant force for social change remains positive.

# References


Abbott, A. (1988) *The System of Professions: an Essay on the Division of Expert Labour*, Chicago: University of Chicago Press.

Adams, J., McCreanor, T. and Braun, V. (2013) 'Gay men's explanations of health and how to improve it', *Qualitative Health Research*, 23(7): 887–899.

Advisory Committee on Breast Cancer Screening (2006) *Screening for Breast Cancer in England: Past and Future*, Sheffield: NHS Screening Programmes.

Alexander, C.E. (2002) 'One of the boys: black masculinity and the peer group' in S. Taylor (ed.) *Ethnographic Research: a Reader*, London: Sage Publications, pp. 91–111.

Alibhai-Brown, Y. (2000) 'Ain't I a woman? The need for a new dialogue about gender and diversity' in A. Coote (ed.) *New Gender Agenda*, London: IPPR, pp. 66–73.

Allen, A. and Hayes, J. (1994) 'Patient satisfaction with telemedicine in a rural clinic', *American Journal of Public Health*, 84(10): 1693.

Allen, D. and Pilnick, A. (2005) 'Making connections: healthcare as a case study in the social organisation of work', *Sociology of Health & Illness*, 27(6): 683–700.

Allsop, J., Jones, K. and Baggott, R. (2004) 'Health consumer groups in the UK: a new social movement?', *Sociology of Health & Illness*, 26: 737–756.

Alvesson, M. and Due Billing, Y. (1997) *Understanding Gender and Organizations*, London: Sage Publications.

Andersson, B. and Ohlen, J. (2005) 'Being a hospice volunteer', *Palliative Medicine*, (19)8: 602–609.

Armstrong, D. (2001) 'From clinical gaze to regime of total health' in T. Heller, R. Muston, M. Sidell and C. Lloyd (eds) *Working for Health*, London: Sage Publications, pp. 16–27.

Armstrong, P. (2010) 'Women's health centres: creating spaces and institutional support' in E. Kuhlmann and E. Annandale (eds) *The Palgrave Handbook of Gender and Healthcare*, Basingstoke: Palgrave Macmillan, pp. 371–386.

Auger, J.A. (2007) 2nd edition *Social Perspectives on Death and Dying*, Halifax, Canada: Fernwood Publishing.

Bach, S., Kessler, I. and Heron, P. (2012) 'Nursing a grievance? The role of healthcare assistants in a modernized National Health Service', *Gender, Work & Organization*, 19(2): 205–224.

Baer, H.A., Singer, M. and Susser, I. (2003) 2nd edition *Medical Anthropology and the World System*, Westport, Connecticut: Praeger Publishers.

Balka, E., Green, E. and Henwood, F. (eds) (2009) *Gender, Health and Information Technology in Context*, Basingstoke: Palgrave Macmillan.

Bakardjieva, M. (2008) 'Virtual togetherness' in J. Johnson and C. De Souza (eds) *Understanding Health and Social Care*, London: Sage Publications and The Open University, pp. 113–119.

Ballard, K.D., Kuh, D.J. and Wadsworth, M.E.J., (2001) 'The role of menopause in women's experiences of the 'change of life'', *Sociology of Health & Illness*, 23: 397–424.

Banks, O. (1981) *Faces of Feminism*, Oxford: Martin Robertson.

Barrett, M. and McIntosh, M. (1982) *The Anti-Social Family*, London: Verso.

Barrow, M. (2013) 'Investing in Online Technology', *Raconteur*, 26 June 2013.

Barry, J., Berg, E. and Chandler, J. (2010) 'The new management of healthcare: "rational" performance and gendered actors' in E. Kuhlmann and E. Annandale (eds) *The Palgrave Handbook of Gender and Healthcare*, Basingstoke: Palgrave Macmillan, pp. 305–320.

Beattie, A. (1991) 'Knowledge and control in health promotion: a test case for social policy and social theory' in J. Gabe, M. Calnan and M. Bury (eds) *The Sociology of the Health Service*, London: Routledge.

Becker, M. (1974) 'The Health Belief Model and personal health behaviour', *Health Education Monographs*, 2(4): 324–473.

Bell, S.E. and Figert, A.E. (2010) 'Gender and the medicalization of healthcare' in E. Kuhlmann and E. Annandale (eds) *Gender and Healthcare*, Basingstoke: Palgrave Macmillan, pp. 107–122.

Bengtsson, T. and van Poppel, F. (2011) 'Socioeconomic inequalities in death from past to present: an introduction', *Explorations in Economic History*, 48(3): 343–356.

Bennett, K.M. (2014) '"I thought I could look after her as good as anybody": how older widowers reconstruct their masculinity' in A. Tarrant and J.H. Watts (eds) *Studies of Ageing Masculinities: Still in their Infancy?*, London: Centre for Policy on Ageing, pp. 20–37.

Bertakis, K.D. and Azari, R. (2007) 'Patient gender and physician practice style', *Journal of Women's Health*, 16(6): 859–868.

Binns, J. (2008) 'The ethics of relational leading: gender matters', *Gender, Work & Organization*, 15(6): 600–620.

Blair-Loy, M. (2004) 'Work devotion and work time' in C.F. Epstein and A.L. Kalleburg (eds) *Fighting for Time: Shifting Boundaries of Work and Social Life*, New York: Russell Sage Foundation, pp. 282–316.

Blow, A.J., Swiecicki, P., Hann, P., Osuch, J.R., Symonds, L.L., Smith, S.S., Walsh, K. and Boivin, M.J. (2011) 'The emotional journey of women experiencing a breast abnormality', *Qualitative Health Research*, 21(10): 1316–1334.

Bolton, S.C. (2005) '"Making up" managers: the case of NHS nurses', *Work, Employment and Society*, 19(1): 5–23.

Bolton, S.C. (2007) 'Gynaecology nursing: dirty work, women's work' in M. Kirkham (ed.) *Exploring the Dirty Side of Women's Health*, London and New York: Routledge, pp. 215–226.

Bolton, S.C. and Houlihan, M. (2009) 'Work, workplaces and workers: the contemporary experience' in S.C. Bolton and M. Houlihan, (eds) *Work Matters: Critical Reflections on Contemporary Work*, Basingstoke: Palgrave Macmillan, pp. 1–20.

Bordo, S. (1993) *Unbearable Weight: Feminism, Western Culture and the Body*, Berkeley, CA: University of California Press.

Boulton, T.N. and Malacrida, C. (2012) 'Women and cosmetic breast surgery: weighing the medical, social and lifestyle risks', *Qualitative Health Research*, 22(4): 511–523.

Broom, A. (2010) 'Prostate cancer and masculinities in Australia' in B. Gough and S. Robertson, (eds) *Men, Masculinities and Health: Critical Perspectives*, Basingstoke: Palgrave Macmillan, pp. 178–197.

Broom, A. and Tovey, P. (eds) (2009) *Men's Health: Body, Identity and Social Context*, London: Wiley-Blackwell.

Broverman, I.K., Broverman, D.M., Clarkson, F.E., Rosenkratz, P.S. and Vogel, S.R. (1970) 'Sex-role stereotypes and clinical judgements of mental health', *Journal of Consulting and Clinical Psychology*, 34(1): 1–7.

Brown, C. and Jones, L. (2004) 'The gender structure of the nursing hierarchy: the role of human capital', *Gender, Work & Organization*, 11(1): 1–25.

Brownmiller, S. (1976) *Against our Will: Men, Women and Rape*, Harmondsworth: Penguin.

Buchbinder, D. (2013) *Studying Men and Masculinities*, Abingdon: Routledge.

Burbeck, R., Low, J., Sampson, L., Bravery, R., Hill, M., Morris, S., Ockenden, N., Payne, S. and Candy, B. (2014) 'Volunteers in specialist palliative care: a survey of adult services in the United Kingdom', *Journal of Palliative Medicine*, 17(10): 1–7.

Burke, R.J. and Nelson, D.L. (2002) 'Advancing women in management: progress and prospects', in R.J. Burke and D.L. Nelson (eds) *Advancing Women's Careers*, Blackwell, Oxford, pp. 3–14.

Burnett, S.B., Gatrell, C.J., Cooper, C.L. and Sparrow, P. (2013) 'Fathers at work: a ghost in the organizational machine', *Gender, Work & Organization*, 20(6): 632–646.

Bury, M. (1982) 'Chronic illness as biographical disruption', *Sociology of Health & Illness*, 4: 167–182.

Busfield, J. (2010) 'Gender and mental health' in E. Kuhlmann and E. Annandale (eds) *Gender and Healthcare*, Basingstoke: Palgrave Macmillan, pp. 172–188.

Butler, J. (1990) *Gender Trouble: Feminism and the Subversion of Identity*, New York: Routledge.

Bytheway, B. and Johnson, J. (2008) 'The social construction of carers' in J. Johnson and C. De Souza (eds) 2nd edition *Understanding Health and Social Care*, London: Sage Publications, pp. 223–232.

Campbell, N.D. and Ettorre, E. (2011) *Gendering Addiction: the Politics of Drug Treatment in a Neurochemical World*, Basingstoke: Palgrave Macmillan.

Cancer Research UK (2004) *Breast Cancer and Breast Screening CancerStats Report*, London: Cancer Research UK.

Carli, L.L. and Eagly, A.H. (2007) 'Overcoming resistance to women leaders: the importance of leadership style' in B. Kellerman and D.L. Rhode (eds) *Women & Leadership*, San Francisco: John Wiley, pp. 127–148.

Carmel, S. and Baker-McClearn, D. (2012) 'Expert nurses and the division of labour in hospitals', *Health*, 16(3): 282–297.

Carpenter, M. (1993) 'The subordination of nurses in health care: towards a social divisions approach' in E. Riska and K. Wegar (eds) *Gender, Work and Medicine: Women and the Medical Division of Labour*, London: Sage Publications, pp. 95–130.

Carrera, M.V., DePalma, R. and Lameiras, M. (2012) 'Sex/gender identity: moving beyond fixed and 'natural' categories', *Sexualities*, 15(8): 995–1016.

Cartwright, L. (1998) 'Community and the public body in breast cancer activism', *Cultural Studies*, 12(2): 117–138.

Cartwright, L. (2000) 'Reach out and heal someone: telemedicine and the globalization of health care', *Health*, 4(3): 347–377.

Cha, Y. (2013) 'Overwork and the persistence of gender segregation in occupations', *Gender & Society*, 27(2): 158–184.

Chaline, E.R. (2010) 'The construction, maintenance and evolution of gay SM sexualities and sexual identities: a preliminary description of gay SM sexual identity practices', *Sexualities*, 13(3): 338–356.

Chancer, L.S. and Watkins, B.X. (2006) *Gender, Race and Class – an Overview*, Malden, MA and Oxford: Blackwell Publishing.

Chapple, A. and McPherson, A. (2004) 'The decision to have a prosthesis: a qualitative study of men with testicular cancer', *Psycho-Oncology*, 13: 654–664.

Chapple, A. and Ziebland, S. (2002) 'Prostate cancer: embodied experience and perceptions of masculinity', *Sociology of Health & Illness*, 24(6): 820–841.

Chapple, A. and Ziebland, S. (2004) 'The role of humour for men with testicular cancer', *Qualitative Health Research*, 14(8): 1123–1139.

Charmaz, K. (1995) 'Identity dilemmas of chronically ill men' in D. Sabo and D.F. Gordon (eds) *Men's Health and Illness: Gender, Power and the Body*, London: Sage Publications, pp. 266–291.

Charteris-Black, J. and Seale, C. (2010) *Gender and the Language of Illness*, Basingstoke: Palgrave Macmillan.

Chesler, P. (1972) *Women and Madness*, London: Allen Lane.

Chodorow, N. (1978) *The Reproduction of Mothering*, Berkeley: University of California Press.

Christie, I. and Jacobs, M. (2000) 'The personal is political (again): a new politics of quality of life' in A. Coote (ed.) *New Gender Agenda*, London: IPPR, pp. 162–179.

Clark, D. and Seymour, J. (1999) *Reflections on Palliative Care*, Buckingham: Open University Press.

Coates, J. (2003) *Men Talk*, Oxford: Blackwell Publishing.

Cockburn, C. (1985) *Machinery of Dominance: Women, Men and Technical Knowhow*, London: Pluto Press.

Colburn, B. (2011) 'Autonomy and adaptive preferences', *Utilitas*, 23: 52–71.

Collinson, D.L. and Collinson, M. (2004) 'The power of time: leadership, management and gender', in C.F. Epstein and A.L. Kalleberg (eds) *Fighting for Time: Shifting Boundaries of Work and Social Life*, Russell Sage Foundation, New York, pp. 219–246.

Coltrane, S. (2008) *Fatherhood, Gender and Work-Family Policies*, available online http://www.ssc.wisc.edu/~mscaglio/2006documents/Coltrane_2007_Fatherhood_Gender_Work-Family.pdf (last accessed 16 December 2013).

Comer, L. (1974) *Wedlocked Women*, Leeds: Feminist Books.

Connell, R.W. (1995) *Masculinities*, Oxford: Polity Press.

Connell, R.W. (2002) *Gender*, Cambridge: Polity Press.

Cook, A. and Glass, C. (2014) 'Women and top leadership positions: towards an institutional analysis', *Gender, Work & Organization*, 21(1): 91–103.

Coontz, S. (2005) *Marriage, a History: from Obedience to Intimacy, or How Love Conquered Marriage*, New York: Viking Press.

Cornwall, A. and Lindisfarne, N. (2005) 'Dislocating masculinity: gender, power and anthropology' in A. Cornwall and N. Lindisfarne (eds) 3rd edition *Dislocating Masculinity*, London and New York: Routledge, pp. 11–47.

Coston, B. and Kimmel, M. (2013) 'Aging men, masculinity and Alzheimer's' in A. Kampf, B.L. Marshall and A. Petersen (eds) *Aging Men. Masculinities and Modern Medicine*, London and New York: Routledge, pp. 191–200.

Cott, N.F. (1986) 'Feminist theory and feminist movements: the past before us' in J. Mitchell and A. Oakley (eds) *What is Feminism?*, Oxford: Basil Blackwell Ltd, pp. 49–62.

Courtenay, W. (2011) *Dying to be Men: Psychosocial, Environmental and Biobehavioural Directions in Promoting the Health of Men and Boys*, London: Routledge.

Cranford, C.J. and Miller, D. (2013) 'Emotion management from the client's perspective: the case of personal home care', *Work, Employment and Society*, 27(5): 785–801.

Cribb, A. (2002) 'Ethics: from health care to public policy' in L. Jones, M. Sidell and J. Douglas (eds) 2nd edition *The Challenge of Promoting Public Health: Exploration and Action*, Basingstoke: Palgrave with The Open University, pp. 261–273.

Crompton, R. (2006) *Employment and the Family*, Cambridge: Cambridge University Press.

Crompton, R. and Lyonette, C. (2011) 'Women's career success and work-life adaptations in the accountancy and medical professions in Britain', *Gender, Work & Organization*, 18(2): 231–254.

Crossley, M.L. (2002) 'The perils of health promotion and the "barebacking" backlash', *Health*, 6(1): 47–68.

Dalley, G. (1996) 2nd edition *Ideologies of Caring*, Basingstoke: Macmillan.

Daly, M. (2002) 'Care as a good for social policy', *Journal of Social Policy*, 31(2): 251–270.

Daniels, C.R. (2001) 'Between fathers and fetuses: the social construction of male reproduction and the politics of fetal harm' in M. Wyer, M. Barbercheck, D. Giesman, H. Orun Ozturk and M. Wayne (eds) *Women, Science and Technology*, New York and London: Routledge, pp. 312–331.

Davies, C. (1995) *Gender and the Professional Predicament in Nursing*, Buckingham: Open University Press.

Davies, K. (2003) 'The body and doing gender: the relations between doctors and nurses in hospital work', *Sociology of Health & Illness*, 25(7): 720–742.

Davis, C.O. (2000) *Death in Abeyance: Illness and Therapy among the Tabwa of Central Africa*, Edinburgh: Edinburgh University Press.

Defellippi, K. and Mnguni, M. (2009) 'Volunteers working in a community palliative care service' in R. Scott and S. Howlett (eds) 2nd edition *Volunteers in Hospice and Palliative Care*, Oxford: Oxford University Press, pp. 177–194.

Dein, S. and Abbas, S.Q. (2005) 'The stresses of volunteering in a hospice: a qualitative study', *Palliative Medicine,* (19)1: 58–64.

DeLaat, J. (1999) *Gender in the Workplace*, London: Sage Publications.

Del Mar Garcia-Calvente, M., Hidalgo-Ruzzante, N., del Rio-Lozano, M., Marcos-Marcos, J., Martinez-Morante, E., Maroto-Navarro, G., Mateo-Rodriguez, I. and Gil-Garcia, E. (2012) 'Exhausted women, tough men: a qualitative study on gender differences in health, vulnerability and coping with illness in Spain', *Sociology of Health & Illness*, 34(6): 911–926.

Delphy, C. (1993) 'Rethinking sex and gender', *Women's Studies International Forum*, 16(1): 1–9.

Dill, B.T. and Kohlman, M.H. (2011) 'Intersectionality: a transformative paradigm in feminist theory and social justice' in S. Hesse-Biber (ed.) 2nd edition *Handbook of Feminist Research*, Thousand Oaks, CA: Sage Publications, pp. 154–174.

Dolan, A. and Coe, C. (2011) 'Men, masculine identities and childbirth', *Sociology of Health & Illness*, 33(7): 1019–1034.

Dolan, A. (2013) '"Men give in to chips and beer too easily": how working-class men make sense of gender differences in health', *Health*, 0(0): 1–17.

Dominelli, L. (2010) *Social Work in a Globalizing World*, Cambridge: Polity Press.

Donnison, J. (1988) 2nd edition *Midwives and Medical Men: A History of the Struggle for the Control of Childbirth*, Barnet, Herts: Historical Publications.

Douglas, M. (2002) Classics edition, *Purity and Danger*, London and New York: Routledge.

Downie, R.S. and Macnaughton, R.J. (1998) 'Images of health', *Lancet*, 351: 823–825.

Downs, M. (2011) 'End of life care for older people with dementia: priorities for research and service development' in M. Gott and C. Ingleton (eds) *Living with Ageing and Dying*, Oxford: Oxford University Press, pp. 247–251.

Doyal, L. (1996) 'The politics of women's health: setting a global agenda', *International Journal of Health Services*, 26(1): 47–65.

Dudgeon, M.R. and Inhorn, M.C. (2003) 'Gender, masculinity and reproduction: anthropological perspectives', *International Journal of Men's Health*, 2(1): 31–56.

Due Billing, Y. (2011) 'Are women in management victims of the phantom of the male norm?', *Gender, Work & Organization*, 18(3): 298–317.

Dyb, K. and Halford, S. (2009) 'Placing globalizing technologies: telemedicine and the making of difference', *Sociology*, 43(2): 232–249.

Dykes, F. (2006) *Breastfeeding in Hospital*, London: Routledge.

Edgell, S. (2006) *The Sociology of Work: Continuity and Change*, London: Sage Publications.

Edwards, J. (2010) 'The healthcare needs of gay and lesbian patients' in E. Kuhlmann, and E. Annandale, (eds) *The Palgrave Handbook of Gender and Healthcare*, Basingstoke: Palgrave Macmillan, pp. 256–271.

Edwards, P. and Wajcman, J. (2005) *The Politics of Working Life*, Oxford: Oxford University Press.

Ehrenreich, B. (2001) 'Welcome to cancerland: a mammogram leads to a cult of pink kitsch', *Harper's Magazine*: 43–53.

Eilberg-Schwartz, H. (1990) *The Savage in Judaism. An Anthropology of Israelite Religion and Ancient Judaism*, Indianapolis: Indiana University Press.

Elson, J. (2004) *Am I Still a Woman? Hysterectomy and Gender Identity*, Philadelphia: Temple University Press.

Emslie, C., Hunt, K. and Watt, G. (2001) 'Invisible women? The importance of gender in lay beliefs about heart problems', *Sociology of Health & Illness*, 23(2): 203–233.

Emslie, C. (2005) 'Women, men and coronary heart disease: a review of the qualitative literature', *Journal of Advanced Nursing*, 51(4): 382–395.

Ettorre, E. and Kingdom, C. (2010) 'Reproductive regimes: governing gendered bodies' in E. Kuhlmann and E. Annandale (eds) *The Palgrave Handbook of Gender and Healthcare*, Basingstoke: Palgrave Macmillan, pp. 142–157.

Evans, M. (2003) *Gender and Social Theory*, Buckingham: Open University Press.

Faludi, S. (1991) *Backlash, The Undeclared War Against Women*, London: Chatto & Windus.

Farrimond, H. (2012) 'Beyond the caveman: rethinking masculinity in relation to men's help-seeking', *Health*, 16(2): 208–225.

Faulkner, A. (2009) *Medical Technology into Healthcare and Society: a Sociology of Devices, Innovation and Governance*, Basingstoke: Palgrave Macmillan.

Faulkner, A. (2012) 'Resisting the screening imperative: patienthood, populations and politics in prostate cancer detection technologies for the UK', *Sociology of Health & Illness*, 34(2): 221–233.

Featherstone, B., Rivett, M. and Scourfield, J. (2007) *Working with Men in Health and Social Care*, London: Sage Publications.

Field, D., Hockey, J. and Small, N. (1997) 'Making sense of difference: death, gender and ethnicity in modern Britain' in D. Field, J. Hockey and N. Small (eds) *Death, Gender and Ethnicity*, London: Routledge, pp. 1–28.

Figes, E. (1970) *Patriarchal Attitudes*, London: Faber.

Fink, J. (2004) 'Questions of care' in J. Fink (ed.) *Care: Personal Lives and Social Policy*, Milton Keynes and Bristol: The Open University and The Policy Press, pp. 1–42.

Firestone, S. (1979) *The Dialectic of Sex*, London: Women's Press.

Fisher, J.R.W., Baker, G.H.W. and Hammarberg, K. (2010) 'Long-term health, well-being, life satisfaction, and attitudes toward parenthood in men diagnosed as infertile: challenges to gender stereotypes and implications for practice', *Fertility and Sterility*, 94(2): 574–580.

Foster, K. (2012) 'Work, narrative identity and social affiliation', *Work, Employment and Society*, 26(6): 935–950.

Foucault, M. (1973) *Birth of the Clinic: An Archaeology of Medical Perception*, London: Tavistock.

Fox, J. (2006) '"Notice how you feel!": an alternative to detached concern among hospice volunteers', *Qualitative Health Research*, 16(7): 944–961.

Frasca, T., Ventuneac, A., Balan, I. and Carballo-Dieguez, A. (2012) 'Inner contradictions among men who bareback', *Qualitative Health Research*, 22(7): 946–956.

Fraser, S. (2004) 'It's your life! Injecting drug users, individual responsibility and hepatitis C prevention', *Health*, 8(2): 199–221.

Freedman, J. (2001) *Feminism*, Buckingham: Open University Press.

Freeman, D. and Freeman, J. (2013) *The Stressed Sex: Uncovering the Truth about Men, Women and Mental Health*, Oxford: Oxford University Press.

Friedan, B. (1963) *The Feminine Mystique*, Harmondsworth: Penguin.

Friedman, S., Sutphen, R. and Steligo, K. (2012) *Confronting Hereditary Breast and Ovarian Cancer*, Baltimore: The John Hopkins University Press.

Freidson, E. (2001) *Professionalism: the Third Logic*, Cambridge: Polity.

Froyum, C.M. (2007) 'At least I am not gay: heterosexual identity making among poor black teens', *Sexualities*, 10(5): 603–622.

Frye, M. (1983) *'Sexism' in the Politics of Reality: Essays in Feminist Theory*, Freedom, California: Crossing Press.

Furedi, A. (2014) 'The barrier to abortion is politics', *Journal of Family Planning & Reproductive Health Care*, 40(1): 5–7.

Galdas, P. (2010) 'The role of masculinities in white and South Asian men's help-seeking behaviour for cardiac chest pain' in B. Gough and S. Robertson (eds) *Men, Masculinities and Health: Critical Perspectives*, Basingstoke: Palgrave Macmillan, pp. 216–231.

Gatrell, C. (2005) *Hard Labour, the Sociology of Motherhood*, Maidenhead: Open University Press.

George, A. (2014) 'Reinventing honorable masculinity: discourses from a working-class Indian community' in J.Z. Spade and C.G. Valentine (eds) 4th edition *The Kaleidoscope of Gender: Prisms, Patterns and Possibilities*, Los Angeles and London: Sage Publications, pp. 138–147.

Gifford, S.M. (2002) 'The meaning of lumps: a case study of the ambiguities of risk' in S. Nettleton and U. Gustafsson (eds) *The Sociology of Health and Illness Reader*, Cambridge: Polity Press, pp. 211–222.

Gilbert, L. and Selikow, T.-A. (2010) 'HIV/AIDS and gender' in E. Kuhlmann and E. Annandale, (eds) *The Palgrave Handbook of Gender and Healthcare*, Basingstoke: Palgrave Macmillan, pp. 189–203.

Gillies, V. (2000) 'Young people and family life: analysing and comparing disciplinary discourses', *Journal of Youth Studies*, 3(2): 211–228.

Gillies, V. (2003) 'Family and intimate relationships: a review of the sociological research', *Families & Social Capital ESRC Research Group Working Paper No. 2*, London South Bank University.

Gilligan, C. (1982) *In a Different Voice*, Cambridge, Mass: Harvard University Press.

Ginsburg, F. (2006) 'Procreation stories: reproduction, nurturance and procreation in life narratives of abortion activists' in E. Lewin (ed.) *Feminist Anthropology*, Oxford: Blackwell Publishing, pp. 235–249.

Goldstein, N.E., Concato, J. and Fried, T.R. (2004) 'Factors associated with caregiver burden among caregivers with terminally ill patients with cancer', *Journal of Palliative Care*, 20(1): 38–43.

Gough, B. and Robertson, S. (eds) (2010) *Men, Masculinities and Health: Critical Perspectives*, Basingstoke: Palgrave Macmillan.

Gottlieb, A. (2002) 'Interpreting gender and sexuality: approaches from cultural anthropology' in J. MacClancy (ed.) *Exotic No More – Anthropology on the Front Line*, Chicago and London: The University of Chicago Press, pp. 167–189.

Graham, H. (2009) *Understanding Health Inequalities*, Maidenhead: Open University Press.

Greener, I. (2007) 'The politics of gender in the NHS: impression management and "getting things done"', *Gender, Work & Organization*, 14(3): 281–299.

Griffiths, F., Bendelow, G., Green, E. and Palmer, J. (2010) 'Screening for breast cancer: medicalization, visualization and the embodied experience', *Health*, 14(6): 653–668.

Grint, K. (2005) 3rd edition *The Sociology of Work*, Cambridge: Polity Press.

Grugulis, I. and Vincent, S. (2009) 'Whose skill is it anyway? "Soft" skills and polarization', *Work Employment and Society*, 23(4): 597–615.

*Guardian*, 15 April 2009 'Young adults delay leaving home: under-35s are increasingly reluctant to fly the nest, statistics show' by John Carvel.

*Guardian*, 3 November 2012 'Barack Obama and the paradox behind his African American support base' by Gary Younge.

Guasp, A. (2011) 'Gay and Bisexual Men's Health Survey', Stonewall www.stonewall.org.uk (accessed 29 August 2014).

Guy, R.A., McDonald, M., Bartlett, J., Murray, C., Geile, T., Davey, R., Appuhamy, P. and Knibbs et al. (2007) 'HIV Diagnoses in Australia: diverging epidemics within a low prevalence country', *Medical Journal of Australia*, 187(8): 437–440.

Hadders, H. (2009) 'Enacting death in the intensive care unit: medical technology and the multiple ontologies of death', *Health*, 13(6): 571–587.

Hadley, R. and Hanley, T. (2011) 'Involuntarily childless men and the desire for fatherhood', *Journal of Reproductive and Infant Psychology*, 29(1): 56–68.

Hakim, C. (2006) 'Women, careers and work-life preferences', *British Journal of Guidance & Counselling*, 34(3): 294–279.

Halford, S., Savage, M. and Witz, A. (1997) *Gender, Careers and Organizations*, Basingstoke: Macmillan Press.

Hallowell, N. (2000) 'Reconstructing the body or reconstructing the woman? Problems of prophylactic mastectomy for hereditary breast cancer risk' in L. Potts (ed.) *Ideologies of Breast Cancer: Feminist Perspectives*, Basingstoke: Macmillan Press, pp. 153–180.

Hanley, R. (2009) 'Volunteers working in a comprehensive palliative care service in Australia' in R. Scott and S. Howlett (eds) 2nd edition *Volunteers in Hospice and Palliative Care*, Oxford: Oxford University Press, pp. 161–176.

Harris, R., Wathen, N. and Wyatt, S. (eds) (2010) *Configuring Health Consumers. Health Work and the Imperative of Personal Responsibility*, Basingstoke: Palgrave Macmillan.

Healy, B. (1991) 'The Yentl Syndrome', *New England Journal of Medicine*, 325(4): 274–276.

Heaphy, B. (2011) 'Gay identities and the culture of class', *Sexualities*, 14(1): 42–62.

Heitman, E. (2002) 'Social and ethical aspects of in vitro fertilization' in S. Nettleton and U. Gustafsson (eds) *The Sociology of Health and Illness Reader*, Cambridge: Polity Press, pp. 57–64.

Hendry, J. (2008) 2nd edition *An Introduction to Social Anthropology*, Basingstoke: Palgrave Macmillan.

Heubel, F. (2000) 'Patents or customers: ethical limits of market economy in health care', *The Journal of Medicine & Philosophy*, 25(2): 240–253.

Higginson, I.J., Finlay, I., Goodwin, D.M., Cook, A.M., Hood, K., Edwards, A.G., Douglas, H.R. and Norman, C.E. (2002) 'Do hospital-based palliative teams improve care for patients or families at the end of life?', *Journal of Pain and Symptom Management*, (23)2: 96–106.

Hippisley-Cox, J., Allen, J., Pringle, M., Ebdon, D., McPhearson, M., Churchill, D. and Bradley, S. (2000) 'Association between teenage pregnancy rates and the age and sex of general practitioners: cross sectional survey in Trent 1994–1997', *British Medical Journal*, 320: 842–845.

Hochschild, A. (1979) 'Emotion work, feeling rules and social structure', *American Journal of Sociology*, 85: 551–575.

Hocquenghem, G. (1972) *Homosexual Desire*, London: Allison & Busby.

Holland, C. (2012) 'The role of technologies in the everyday lives of older people' in J. Katz, S. Peace and S. Spurr (eds) *Adult Lives – a Life Course Perspective*, Bristol: Policy Press with the Open University, pp. 151–160.

Holmes, M. (2009) *Gender and Everyday Life*, London and New York: Routledge.

Holt, M. and Stephenson, N. (2006) 'Living with HIV and negotiating psychological discourse', *Health*, 10(2): 211–231.

hooks, b. (2000) *Where we Stand: Class Matters*, New York: Routledge.

hooks, b. (2013) *Writing Beyond Race: Living Theory and Practice*, New York and London: Routledge.

Howard, S. and Welbourn, D. (2004) *The Spirit at Work Phenomenon*, London: Azure.

Howlett, S. (2009) 'Setting the scene: the landscape of volunteering' in R. Scott and S. Howlett (eds) 2nd edition *Volunteers in Hospice and Palliative Care*, Oxford: Oxford University Press, pp. 11–19.

Hubbard, R. and Wald, E. (1997) *Exploding the Gene Myth*, Boston, MA: Beacon Press.

Hughes, A. (2010) 'The challenge of contributing to policy making in primary care: the gendered experiences and strategies of nurses', *Sociology of Health & Illness*, 32(7): 977–992.

Hurrell, S.A., Scholarios, D. and Thompson, P. (2013) 'More than a "humpty dumpty" term: strengthening the conceptualization of soft skills', *Economic and Industrial Democracy*, 34(1): 161–182.

Jackson, D. (2014) 'Ageing men are changing men: emancipatory possibilities for ageing men' in A. Tarrant and J. H. Watts (eds) *Studies of Ageing Masculinities: Still in their Infancy?*, London: Centre for Policy on Ageing, pp. 55–67.

Jackson, S. and Scott, S. (2002) 'Introduction' in S. Jackson and S. Scott (eds) *Gender: a Sociological Reader*, London and New York: Routledge, pp. 1–26.

Jaworski, K. (2014) *The Gender of Suicide: Knowledge Production, Theory and Suicidology*, Farnham: Ashgate.

Johnson, J.L., Oliffe, J.L., Kelly, M.T., Galdas, P. and Ogrodniczuk, J.S. (2012) 'Men's discourses of help-seeking in the context of depression', *Sociology of Health & Illness*, 34(3): 345–361.

Johnson, K.M. and Simon, R.M. (2012) 'Women's attitudes toward biomedical technology for infertility: the case for technological salience', *Gender & Society*, 26(2): 261–289.

Kampf, A. (2013) 'Tales of healthy men: male reproductive bodies in biomedicine from 'Lebensborn' to sperm banks', *Health*, 17(1): 20–36.

Karlsen, H. (2012) 'Gender and ethnic differences in occupational positions and earnings among nurses and engineers in Norway: identical educational choices, unequal outcomes', *Work, Employment and Society*, 26(2): 278–295.

Kaufman, S.R. (2005) *And a Time to Die: How American Hospitals Shape the End of Life*, Chicago: The University of Chicago Press.

Kearney, A.J. (2006) 'Increasing our understanding of breast self-examination: women talk about cancer, the healthcare system, and being women', *Qualitative Health Research*, 16(6): 802–820.

Kellehear, A. (1994) 'The social inequality of dying' in C. Waddell and A.R. Petersen (eds) *Just Health: Inequality in Illness, Care and Prevention*, Melbourne: Churchill Livingstone, pp. 181–189.

Kellehear, A. (2007) *A Social History of Dying*, New York: Cambridge University Press.

Kellehear, A. (2012) 'The importance of family carers in end-of-life care: a public health approach' in J. Cohen and L. Deliens (eds) *A Public Health Perspective on End of Life Care*, Oxford: Oxford University Press, pp. 227–238.

Kelly, D. (2009) 'Changed men: the embodied impact of prostate cancer', *Qualitative Health Research*, 19(2): 151–163.

Khader, S.J. (2011) *Adaptive Preferences and Women's Empowerment*, Oxford: Oxford University Press.

Klaeson, K., Sandell, K. and Bertero, C.M. (2012) 'Sexuality in the context of prostate cancer narratives', *Qualitative Health Research*, 22(9): 1184–1194.

Kolip, P. (2010) 'Primary prevention and health promotion: towards gender-sensitive interventions' in E. Kuhlmann and E. Annandale (eds) *The Palgrave Handbook of Gender and Healthcare*, Basingstoke: Palgrave Macmillan, pp. 337–354.

Kontos, P.C. (2010) 'Embodied selfhood: ethnographic reflections, performing ethnography and humanizing dementia care' in J.E. Graham and P.H. Stephenson (eds) *Contesting Aging & Loss*, Toronto: University of Toronto Press, pp. 125–152.

Kottak, C.P. (2004) 10th edition *Cultural Anthropology*, New York: McGraw-Hill.

Kuhlmann, E. and Annandale, E. (eds) (2010) *The Palgrave Handbook of Gender and Healthcare*, Basingstoke: Palgrave Macmillan.

Kumra, S. and Vinnicombe, S. (2010) 'Impressing for success: a gendered analysis of a key social accumulation strategy', *Gender, Work & Organization*, 17(5): 521–546.

Lagro-Janssen, T. (2010) 'Sex, gender and health: developments in medical research' in E. Kuhlmann and E. Annandale (eds) (2010) *The Palgrave Handbook of Gender and Healthcare*, Basingstoke: Palgrave Macmillan, pp. 405–420.

Larkin, P. and Hegarty, M. (2011) 'Workforce development: an international perspective on who will provide care' in M. Gott and C. Ingleton (eds) *Living with Ageing and Dying*, Oxford: Oxford University Press, pp. 191–201.

Laverack, G. (2014) *A-Z of Health Promotion*, Basingstoke: Palgrave Macmillan.

Lean, S. and McDermott, P. (2009) 'Professionals working as volunteers' in R. Scott and S. Howlett (eds) 2nd edition *Volunteers in Hospice and Palliative Care*, Oxford: Oxford University Press, pp. 109–118.

Lewis, P. and Simpson, R. (2010) 'Introduction: theoretical insights into the practices of revealing and concealing gender within organizations' in P. Lewis and R. Simpson (eds) *Revealing and Concealing Gender: Issues of Visibility in Organizations*, Basingstoke: Palgrave Macmillan, pp. 1–22.

Lewis, S. (2002) 'Work and family issues: old and new' in R.J. Burke and D.L. Nelson (eds) *Advancing Women's Careers*, Oxford: Blackwell Publishing, pp. 67–82.

Lewis, S. (2014) 'Could generalists lead the war against excess in the NHS?', *Guardian Professional*, accessed online: www.guardian.com/healthcare-network, 6 March 2014.

Liamputtong, P., Haritavom, N. and Kiatying-Angsulee, N. (2012) 'Living positively: the experiences of Thai women living with HIV/AIDS in central Thailand', *Qualitative Health Research*, 22(4): 441–451.

Lindsay, S. (2008) 'The care-tech link: an examination of gender, care and technical work in healthcare labour', *Gender, Work & Organization*, 15(4): 333–351.

Lips, H.M. (2014) *Gender: the Basics*, London and New York: Routledge.

Lister, R. (1997) *Citizenship: Feminist Perspectives*, Basingstoke: Macmillan Press.

Lock, M. (2002) 'Medical knowledge and body politics' in J. MacClancy (ed.) *Exotic No More: Anthropology on the Front Lines*, London: The University of Chicago Press, pp. 190–208.

Loe, M. (2010) 'Doing it my way: old women, technology and wellbeing', *Sociology of Health & Illness*, 32(2): 319–334.

Lorber, J. (1984) *Women Physicians*, London: Tavistock.

Lupton, D. (2002) 'Consumerism, reflexivity and the medical encounter' in S. Nettleton and U. Gustafsson (eds) *The Sociology of Health and Illness Reader*, Cambridge: Polity Press, pp. 360–368.

Macintyre, S., MacIver, S. and Sooman, A. (2002) 'Area, class and health: should we be focusing on places or people?' in S. Nettleton and U. Gustafsson (eds) *The Sociology of Health and Illness Reader*, Cambridge: Polity Press, pp. 278–292.

Magnusson, C. (2010) 'Why is there a gender wage gap according to occupational prestige?', *Acta Sociologica*, 53(2): 99–117.

Martin, G.P. (2007) '"Ordinary people only": knowledge, representativeness, and the publics of public participation in healthcare', *Sociology of Health & Illness*, 30: 35–54.

Martin, L.J. (2010) 'Anticipating infertility: egg freezing, genetic preservation and risk', *Gender & Society*, 24(4): 526–545.

Martin, G.P. and Finn, R. (2011) 'Patients as team members: opportunities, challenges and paradoxes of including patients in multi-professional healthcare teams', *Sociology of Health & Illness*, 33: 1050–1065.

Martin, G.P. and Waring, J. (2013) 'Leading from the middle: constrained realities of clinical leadership in healthcare organizations', *Health*, 17(4): 358–374.

Matthews, J. (1984) *Good and Mad Women: the Historical Construction of Femininity in Twentieth Century Australia*, Sydney: George Allen and Unwin.

Maushart, S. (2002) *Wifework: What Marriage Really Means for Women*, London: Bloomsbury.

May, C. and Ellis, N. (2001) 'When protocols fail: technical evaluation, biomedical knowledge and the social production of "facts" about a telemedicine clinic', *Social Science and Medicine*, 53(8): 989–1002.

Mckenna, H.P., Hasson, F. and Keeney, S. (2004) 'Patient safety and quality of care: the role of the health care assistant', *Journal of Nursing Management*, 12: 452–459.

McLaughlin, K., Muldoon, O.T. and Moutray, M. (2010) 'Gender, gender roles and completion of nursing education: a longitudinal study', *Nurse Education Today*, 30: 303–307.

Mead, M. (1935) *Sex and Temperament in Three Primitive Societies*, New York: Harper Collins.

Miller, W.I. (2011) *Losing It*, New Haven and London: Yale University Press.

Millett, K. (1970) *Sexual Politics*, London: Abacus/Sphere.

Mitchell, J. (1971) *Women's Estate*, Harmondsworth: Penguin.

Mooney, G. (2004) 'Exploring the dynamics of work, personal lives and social policy' in G. Mooney (ed.) *Work, Personal Lives and Social Policy*, Milton Keynes and Bristol: The Open University and The Policy Press, pp. 1–38.

Mooney, J. (2000) *Gender, Violence and the Social Order*, Basingstoke: Palgrave Macmillan.

Moore, S. (2009) '"No matter what I did I would still end up in the same position": age as a factor defining older women's experience of labour market participation', *Work, Employment and Society*, 23(4): 655–671.

Moore, G. (2014) 'Mommies and daddies on the fast track in other wealthy nations' in J.Z. Spade and C.G. Valentine (eds) 4th edition *The Kaleidoscope of Gender: Prisms, Patterns and Possibilities*, London: Sage Publications, pp. 387–398.

Morgan, D. (1993) 'You too can have a body like mine: reflections on the male body and masculinities' in S. Scott and D. Morgan (eds) *Body Matters: Essays on the Sociology of the Body*, London: Falmer Press.

Morgan, J.C., Dill, J. and Kalleberg, A.L. (2013) 'The quality of healthcare jobs: can intrinsic rewards compensate for low extrinsic rewards?', *Work Employment and Society*, 27(5): 802–822.

Morgan, R. (1970) (ed.) *Sisterhood is Powerful*, New York: Vantage Books.

Morris, L. (1999) 'Work, gender and unemployment: a household perspective' in S. Walby (ed.) *New Agendas for Women*, Basingstoke, Macmillan Press, pp. 32–44.

Muzio, D. and Bolton, S.C. (2006) 'Feminisation and paradox: stratification and segmentation in professional contexts', *The Irish Journal of Management*, 1: 79–93.

Naidoo, J. and Wills, J. (2009) 3rd edition *Health Promotion: Foundations for Practice*, London: Saunders.

Nettleton, S. and Gustafsson, U. (2002) 'Introduction' in S. Nettleton and U. Gustafsson (eds) *The Sociology of Health and Illness Reader*, Cambridge: Polity Press, pp. 1–10.

Newman, J. and Mooney, G. (2004) 'Managing personal lives: doing "welfare work"' in G. Mooney (ed.) *Work: Personal Lives and Social Policy*, Milton Keynes and Bristol: The Open University and The Policy Press, pp. 39–72.

Nicholson, C. and Hockley, J. (2011) 'Death and dying in older people' in D. Oliviere, B. Monroe and S. Payne (eds) 2nd edition *Death, Dying and Social Differences*, Oxford: Oxford University Press, pp. 101–109.

Noon, M. and Blyton, P. (2007) *The Realities of Work: Experiencing Work and Employment in Contemporary Society*, Basingstoke: Palgrave Macmillan.

Noone, J.H. and Stephens, C. (2008) 'Men, masculine identities and health care utilisation', *Sociology of Health & Illness*, 30(5): 711–725.

Nosek, M., Kennedy, H.P. and Gudmundsdottir, M. (2012) '"Chaos, restitution and quest": one woman's journey through menopause', *Sociology of Health & Illness*, 34(7): 994–1009.

Oakley, A. (1972) *Sex, Gender and Society*, London: Temple Smith.

Oakley, A. (1974) *The Sociology of Housework*, London: Martin Robertson.

Oakley, A. (1976) *Housewife: High Value, Low Cost*, London: Penguin.

Oakley, A. (1984) *The Captured Womb: A History of the Medical Care of Pregnant Women*, Oxford: Basil Blackwell.

Oakley, A. (1986) 'Feminism, motherhood and medicine – who cares?' in J. Mitchell and A. Oakley (eds) *What is Feminism?*, Oxford: Basil Blackwell, pp. 127–150.

Oakley, A. (1987) 'From walking wombs to test-tube babies' in M. Stanworth (ed.) *Reproductive Technologies: Gender, Motherhood and Medicine*, Cambridge: Polity Press, pp. 36–56.

O'Connor, M. and Gwyther, L. (2014) 'Strengthening international networks to advance global palliative care', *Illness, Crisis & Loss*, 22(1): 3–10.

Oliviere, D. and Monroe, B. (2004) 'Introduction: working with death, dying and difference' in D. Oliviere and B. Monroe (eds) *Death, Dying and Social Differences*, Oxford: Oxford University Press, pp. 1–5.

ONS, Office for National Statistics (2011) *Colorectal Cancer in England, 2008*, http://www.ons.gov.uk.

ONS, Office for National Statistics (2012) *Death Registrations by Single Year of Age – United kingdom, 2011*, http://www.ons.gov.uk.

Ortner, S. (1974) 'Is female to male as nature is to culture?' in M.Z. Rosaldo and L. Lamphere (eds) *Women, Culture and Society*, Stanford, California: Stanford University Press, pp. 67–87.

Osterfield, J. (2009) 'Volunteers working in a bereavement service' in R. Scott and S. Howlett (eds) 2nd edition *Volunteers in Hospice and Palliative Care*, Oxford: Oxford University Press, pp. 131–143.

Oudshoorn, N. (2011) *Telecare Technologies and the Transformation of Healthcare*, Basingstoke: Palgrave Macmillan.

Palmer, E. and Eveline, J. (2012) 'Sustaining low pay in aged care work', *Gender, Work & Organization*, 19(3): 254–275.

Parsons, T. and Bales, R. (1956) *Family and Socialisation and Interaction Process*, London: Routledge and Kegan Paul.

Pas, B., Peters, P., Elsinga, R., Doorewaard, H. and Lagro-Janssen, T. (2011) 'Explaining career motivation among female doctors in the Netherlands: the effects of children, views on motherhood and work-home cultures', *Work, Employment and Society*, 25(3): 487–505.

Pascall, G. (1997) *Social Policy: a New Feminist Analysis*, London and New York: Routledge.

Pateman, C. (1988) *The Sexual Contract*, Cambridge: Polity Press.

Pavis, S., Cunningham-Burley, S. and Amos, A. (2002) 'Health related behavioural change in context: young people in transition' in S. Nettleton and U. Gustafsson (eds) *The Sociology of Health and Illness Reader*, Cambridge, Polity Press, pp. 119–132.

Payne. S. (2004) 'Carers and caregivers' in D. Oliviere and B. Monroe (eds) *Death, Dying and Social Differences*, Oxford: Oxford University Press, pp. 181–198.

Payne, S. (2006) *The Health of Men and Women*, Cambridge: Policy Press.

Penner, A.M. and Saperstein, A. (2013) 'Engendering racial perceptions: an intersectional analysis of how social status shapes race', *Gender & Society*, 27(3): 319–344.

Peronace, L.A., Boivin, J. and Schmidt, L. (2007) 'Patterns of suffering and social interactions in infertile men: 12 months after unsuccessful treatment', *Journal of Psychosomatic Obstetrics & Gynecology*, 28(2): 105–114.

Picardie, R. (1998) *Before I Say Goodbye*, London: Penguin.

Pichardo, J.I. (2011) 'We are family (or not): social and legal recognition of same-sex relationships and lesbian and gay families in Spain', *Sexualities*, 14(5): 544–561.

Pietila, I. and Rytkonen, M. (2008) '"Health is not a man's domain". Lay accounts of gender difference in life-expectancy in Russia', *Sociology of Health & Illness*, 30(7): 1070–1085.

Pilcher, J. and Whelan, I. (2004) *50 Key Concepts in Gender Studies*, London: Sage Publications.

Pinquart, M. and Sorensen, S. (2003) 'Differences between caregivers and noncaregivers in psychological health and physical health: a meta-analysis', *Psychology and Aging*, 18: 250–267.

Porter, R. (1999) *A Medical History of Humanity from Antiquity to the Present*, London: Fontana.

Potts, L. (2000) 'Introduction: why ideologies of breast cancer? Why feminist perspectives?', in L. Potts (ed.) *Ideologies of Breast Cancer: Feminist Perspectives*, Basingstoke: Macmillan Press, pp. 1–11.

Powell, G.N. (1999) 'Reflections on the glass ceiling: recent trends and future prospects' in G.N. Powell (ed.) *Handbook of Gender and Work*, Thousand Oaks, CA: Sage Publications, pp. 325–345.

Pratchett, T. (2011) 'Living with early dementia' in C. Lloyd and T. Heller (eds) *Long-term Conditions: Challenges in Health and Social Care*, London: Sage Publications, pp. 5–9.

Price-Glynn, K. and Rakovski, C. (2012) 'Who rides the glass escalator? Gender, race and nationality in the national nursing assistant survey', *Work, Employment and Society*, 26(5): 699–715.

Prior, L. (2003) 'Belief, knowledge and expertise: the emergence of the lay expert in medical sociology', *Sociology of Health & Illness*, 25: 41–57.

Pyke, K.D. (1996) 'Class-based masculinities: the interdependence of gender, class and interpersonal power', *Gender & Society*, 10: 527–549.

Pyper, C., Amery, J., Watson, M. and Cook, C. (2004) 'Patients' experiences of accessing their electronic patient records', *British Journal of General Practice*, 54: 38–43.

Rabinovitch, D. (2007) *Take Off Your Party Dress*, London: Pocket Books.

Randall, F. and Downie, R.S. (2006) *The Philosophy of Palliative Care: Critique and Reconstruction*, Oxford: Oxford University Press.

Rapport, F., Doel, M.A., Greaves, D. and Elwyn, G. (2006) 'From manila to monitor: biographies of general practitioner workspaces', *Health*, 10(2): 233–251.

Reed, K. (2013) 'Beyond hegemonic masculinity: the role of family genetic history in men's accounts of health', *Sociology*, 47(5): 906–920.

Reeve, J., Lloyd-Williams, M., Payne, S. and Dowrick, C. (2010) 'Revisiting biographical disruption: exploring individual embodied illness experience in people with terminal cancer', *Health*, 14(2): 178–195.

Rendall, J. (1990) *Women in an Industrializing Society: England 1750-1880*, Oxford: Blackwell.

Rich, A. (1976) *Of Woman Born: Motherhood as Experience and Institution*, New York: W. W. Norton.

Ridge, D., Emslie, C. and White, A. (2011) 'Understanding how men experience, express and cope with mental distress: where next?', *Sociology of Health & Illness*, 33(1): 145–159.

Riska, E. (1993) 'Introduction' in E. Riska and K. Wegar (eds) *Gender, Work and Medicine*, London: Sage Publications, pp. 1–12.

Riska, E. (2002) 'From type A man to the hardy man: masculinity and health', *Sociology of Health & Illness*, 24(3): 347–358.

Riska, E. (2010a) 'Women in the medical profession: international trends' in E. Kuhlmann and E. Annandale (eds) *The Palgrave Handbook of Gender and Healthcare*, Basingstoke: Palgrave Macmillan, pp. 389–404.

Riska, E. (2010b) 'Coronary heart disease: gendered public health discourses' in E. Kuhlmann and E. Annandale (eds) *The Palgrave Handbook of Gender and Healthcare*, Basingstoke: Palgrave Macmillan, pp. 158–171.

Roberts, D.E. (2014) 'Race, gender and genetic technologies: a new reproductive dystopia?' in M. Wyer, M. Barbercheck, D. Cookmeyer, H.O. Ozturk and M. Wayne (eds) 3rd edition *Women, Science, and Technology: a Reader in Feminist Science Studies*, New York: Routledge, pp. 318–333.

Robertson, S. (2007) *Understanding Men and Health*, Maidenhead: Open University Press.

Robertson, S., Sheikh, K. and Moore, A. (2010) 'Embodied masculinities in the context of cardiac rehabilitation', *Sociology of Health & Illness*, 32(5): 695–710.

Robinson, V. and Hockey, J. (2011) *Masculinities in Transition*, Basingstoke: Palgrave Macmillan.

Rogers, A. and Pilgrim, D. (2005) 3rd edition *The Sociology of Mental Health and Illness*, Maidenhead: Open University Press.

Rose, H. (1987) 'Victorian values in the test-tube: the politics of reproductive science and technology' in M. Stanworth (ed.) *Reproductive Technologies: Gender, Motherhood and Medicine*, Cambridge: Polity Press, pp. 151–173.

Rose, H. (1994) *Love, Power and Knowledge*, Cambridge: Polity Press.

Rose, N. (2010) 'Normality and pathology in a biomedical age', *The Sociological Review*, 57: 66–83.

Rose, H. and Bruce, E. (1995) 'Mutual care but differential esteem: caring between older couples' in S. Arber and J. Ginn (eds) *Connecting Gender and Ageing*, Buckingham: Open University Press, pp. 114–129.

Ryle, R. (2012) *Questioning Gender: a Sociological Exploration*, London: Sage Publications.

Saltonstall, R. (1993) 'Healthy bodies, social bodies: men's and women's concepts and practices of health in everyday life', *Social Science and Medicine*, 36(1): 7–14.

Sandman, L. (2005) *A Good Death: On the Value of Death and Dying*, Maidenhead: Open University Press.

Saul, J.M. (2003) *Feminisms: Issues & Arguments*, Oxford: Oxford University Press.

Saywell, C., Beattie, L. and Henderson, L. (2000) 'Sexualised illness: the newsworthy body in media representations of breast cancer' in L. Potts (ed.) *Ideologies of Breast Cancer: Feminist Perspectives*, Basingstoke: Macmillan Press, pp. 37–62.

Schmidt, J. (2003) 'Paradise lost? Social change and fa'afafine in Samoa', *Current Sociology*, 51(3/4): 417–432.

Schneiderman, L.J. and Jecker, N.S. (2011) 2nd edition *Wrong Medicine: Doctors, Patients and Futile Treatment*, Baltimore: The John Hopkins University Press.

Schofield, T. (2010) 'Men's health and well-being' in E. Kuhlmann and E. Annandale (eds) *The Palgrave Handbook of Gender and Healthcare*, Basingstoke: Palgrave Macmillan, pp. 239–255.

Segal, L. (1990) *Slow Motion: Changing Masculinities Changing Men*, London: Virago Press.

Segal, L. (1999) *Why Feminism?*, Cambridge: Polity Press.

Segal, L. (2013) *Out of Time*, London and New York: Verso.

Serra, H. (2010) 'Medical technocracies in liver transplantation: drawing boundaries in medical practices', *Health*, 14(2): 162–177.

Sheaff, M. (2005) *Sociology and Health Care*, Maidenhead: Open University Press.

Sheff, E. (2006) 'Poly-hegemonic masculinities', *Sexualities*, 9(5): 621–642.

Sidell, M. (2001) 'Understanding chronic illness' in T. Heller, R. Muston, M. Sidell and C. Lloyd (eds) *Working for Health*, London: Sage Publications, pp. 255–265.

Silva, E.B. (1999) 'Transforming Housewifery: dispositions, practices and technologies' in E.B. Silva and C. Smart (eds) *The New Family?*, London: Sage Publications, pp. 46–65.

Silva, E.B. and Smart, C. (1999) 'The 'new' practices and politics of family life' in E.B. Silva and C. Smart (eds) *The New Family?*, London: Sage Publications, pp. 1–12.

Simpson, C. (2000) 'Controversies in breast cancer prevention: the discourse of risk' in L. Potts (ed.) *Ideologies of Breast Cancer: Feminist Perspectives*, Basingstoke: Macmillan Press, pp. 131–152.

Simpson, R. (2009) *Men in Caring Occupations: Doing Gender Differently*, Basingstoke: Palgrave Macmillan.

Sinclair, P. (2007) *Rethinking Palliative Care*, Bristol: The Policy Press.

Skeggs, B. (1997) *Formations of Class and Gender*, London: Sage Publications.

Small, N. and Sargeant, A. (2011) 'User and community participation at the end of life' in M. Gott and C. Ingleton (eds) *Living with Ageing and Dying*, Oxford: Oxford University Press, pp. 90–101.

Smith, A.M. (1992) 'Resisting the erasure of lesbian sexuality: a challenge for queer activism' in K. Plummer (ed.) *Modern Homosexualities: Fragments of Lesbian and Gay Experience*, London: Routledge.

Smith, D.E. (1974) 'Women's perspective as a radical critique of sociology', *Sociological Inquiry*, 44(1): 7–13.

Spector-Mersel, G. (2006) 'Never-aging stories: Western hegemonic masculinity scripts', *Journal of Gender Studies*, 15(1): 67–82.

Spender, D. (1985) *For the Record*, London: The Women's Press.

Stacey, J. (1997) 'Feminist theory: capital F, capital T' in V. Robinson and D. Richardson (eds) 2nd edition *Introducing Women's Studies*, London: Macmillan.

Stacey, J. (2006) 'Gay parenthood and the decline of paternity as we knew it', *Sexualities*, 9(1): 27–55.

Stajduhar, K.I. (2011) 'Family carers and social difference' in D. Oliviere, B. Monroe and S. Payne (eds) 2nd edition *Death, Dying and Social Differences*, Oxford: Oxford University Press, pp. 183–190.

Stanko, E. (1988) 'Keeping women in and out of line: sexual harassment and occupational segregation' in S. Walby (ed.) *Gender Segregation at Work*, Milton Keynes: Open University Press.

Stanley, L. and Wise, S. (1993) 2nd edition *Breaking Out Again – Feminist Ontology and Epistemology*, London: Routledge.

Stanworth, M. (1987) (ed.) *Reproductive Technologies: Gender, Motherhood and Medicine*, Cambridge: Polity Press.

Stebbins, R.A. (1996) 'Volunteering: a serious leisure perspective', *Nonprofit and Voluntary Sector Quarterly*, 25(2): 211–224.

Stokowski, L.A. (2012) 'Just call us nurses: men in nursing', *Medscape*, 16 August 2012.

Sulik, G.A. (2007) 'The balancing act: care work for the self and coping with breast cancer', *Gender & Society*, 21(6): 857–877.

Sulik, G.A. (2012) *Pink Ribbon Blues: How Breast Cancer Culture Undermines Women's Health*, Oxford: Oxford University Press.

Szewczuk, E. (2012) 'Age-related infertility: a tale of two technologies', *Sociology of Health & Illness*, 34(3): 429–443.

Tadel, P.M. (2014) 'Wading in the water: a case study approach to engaging more fully in the patient narrative', *Illness, Crisis & Loss*, 22(1): 11–27.

Taylor, D. and Bury, M. (2007) 'Chronic illness, expert patients and care transition', *Sociology of Health & Illness*, 29(1): 27–45.

Thomas, C. (1999) *Female Forms: Experiencing and Understanding Disability*, Buckingham: Open University Press.

Thompson, C. (2006) 'Strategic naturalizing: kinship in an infertility clinic' in E. Lewin (ed.) *Feminist Anthropology*, Oxford: Blackwell Publishing, pp. 271–288.

Thompson, L., Reeder, T. and Abel, G. (2012) '"I can't get my husband to go and have a colonoscopy": gender and screening for colorectal cancer', *Health*, 16(3): 235–249.

Throsby, K. and Gill, R. (2004) '"It's different for men": masculinity and IVF', *Men and Masculinities*, 6(4): 330–348.

Timmons, S. and East, L. (2011) 'Uniforms, status and professional boundaries in hospital', *Sociology of Health & Illness*, 33(7): 1035–1049.

Travis, C.B., Meltzer, A.I. and Howerton, D.M. (2010) 'Gender issues in health care utilization' in J. Chrisler and D.R. McCreary (eds) *Handbook of Gender Research in Psychology (Vol 2)*, New York: Springer, pp. 517–540.

Turner, B. (2004) *The New Medical Sociology: Social Forms of Health and Illness*, New York and London: W. W. Norton & Company.

Twomey, M. (2012) 'Autonomy and reason: treatment choice in breast cancer', *Journal of Evaluation in Clinical Practice*, 18(5): 1045–1050.

Ugreninov, E. (2013) 'Offspring in squeeze: health and sick leave absence among middle-aged informal caregivers', *Population Ageing*, 6: 323–338.

Vinnicombe, S. and Singh, V. (2002) 'Developing tomorrow's women business leaders' in R.J. Burke and D.L. Nelson (eds) *Advancing Women's Careers*, Oxford: Blackwell, pp. 206–219.

Wajcman, J. (1991) *Feminism Confronts Technology*, Philadelphia, PA: Penn State University Press.

Wajcman, J. (1998) *Managing like a Man: Women and Men in Corporate Management*, Cambridge: Polity Press.

Wajcman, J. (2000) 'Reflections on gender and technology studies', *Social Studies of Science*, 3(3): 447–464.

Walby, S. (1986) *Patriarchy at Work*, Oxford: Polity Press.

Walby, S. (1990) *Theorizing Patriarchy*, Oxford: Blackwell.

Walby, S. (2011) *The Future of Feminism*, Cambridge: Polity Press.

Walby, S., Armstrong, J. and Strid, S. (2012) 'Intersectionality: multiple inequalities in social theory', *Work, Employment and Society*, 46(2): 224–240.

Wallace, J.E. (2014) 'Gender and supportive co-worker relations in the medical profession', *Gender, Work & Organization*, 21(1): 1–17.

Walsh, J. (2013) 'Gender, the work-life interface and wellbeing: a study of hospital doctors', *Gender, Work & Organization*, 20(4): 439–453.

Walter, T. (2003) 'Historical and cultural variants on the good death', *British Medical Journal*, 327: 218–220.

Wangui, E.E. (2009) 'Livelihood strategies and nutritional status of grandparent caregivers of AIDS orphans in Nyando district, Kenya', *Qualitative Health Research*, 19(12): 1702–1715.

Warren, T. (2007) 'Conceptualising breadwinning work', *Work, Employment and Society*, 21(2): 317–336.

Warwick-Booth, L., Cross, R. and Lowcock, D. (2012) *Contemporary Health Studies: an Introduction*, Cambridge: Polity Press.

Watts, J.H. (2007a) 'Porn, pride and pessimism: experiences of women working in professional construction roles', *Work, Employment and Society*, 21 (2): 297–314.

Watts, J. (2007b) 'Can't take a joke? Humour as resistance, refuge and exclusion in a highly gendered workplace'. *Feminism & Psychology*, 17 (2): 259–266.

Watts, J.H. (2007c) 'Allowed into a man's world'. Meanings of work/life balance: perspectives of women civil engineers as minority workers in construction. *Gender Work & Organization*, On-Line Early.

Watts, J.H. (2008) 'Impression management: a form of emotion work for women in a male-dominated profession', *International Journal of Work Organization and Emotion*, 2 (3): 221–235.

Watts, J.H. (2009) 'Leaders of men: women "managing" in construction', *Work, Employment and Society*, 23(3): 512–530.

Watts, J.H. (2010) *Death, Dying and Bereavement: Issues for Practice*, Edinburgh: Dunedin Academic Press.

Watts, J.H. (2012) 'Working as a hospice volunteer', *Illness Crisis & Loss*, 20(2): 101–117.

West, C. and Zimmerman, D.H. (1987) 'Doing gender', *Gender & Society*, 1(2): 125–151.

Whitehead, S. (2002) *Men and Masculinities*, Cambridge: Polity Press.

Whittock, M., Edwards, C., McLaren, S. and Robinson. O. (2002) 'The tender trap: gender, part-time nursing and the effects of "family-friendly" policies on career advancement', *Sociology of Health & Illness*, 24(3): 305–326.

WHO, World Health Organisation (1985) *Targets for Health for All*, Geneva: WHO.

WHO, World Health Organisation (2002) National Cancer Control Programmes: Policies and Managerial Guidelines, 2nd edition, Geneva: WHO.

WHO, World Health Organisation (2005) *The Bangkok Charter for Health Promotion in a Globalised World*, Geneva: WHO.

WHO, World Health Organisation (2013) *Global Health Observatory: NCD Mortality and Morbidity*, Geneva: WHO.

Williams, F. (2004) *Rethinking Families*, London: Calouste Gulbenkian Foundation.

Williams, J. (2000) *Unbending Gender: Why Family and Work Conflict and What to do About it*, Oxford: Oxford University Press.

Wilson, D.M. and Mohankumar, D. (2012) 'End-of-life care for people who live in rural or remote areas versus those who live in urban areas' in J. Cohen and L. Deliens (eds) *A Public Health Perspective on End of Life Care*, Oxford: Oxford University Press, pp. 178–182.

Wingfield, A.H. (2014) 'Racialising the glass escalator: reconsidering men's experiences with women's work' in J.Z. Spade and C.G. Valentine (eds) 4th edition *The Kaleidoscope of Gender: Prisms, Patterns and Possibilities*, London: Sage Publications, pp. 366–376.

Woods, B. and Pratt, R. (2005) 'Awareness in dementia: ethical and legal issues in relation to people with dementia', *Aging & Mental Health*, 9(5): 423–429.

Woods, S. (2007) *Death's Dominion: Ethics at the End of Life*, Maidenhead: Open University Press.

Woodward, K. (ed.) (1997) *Identity and Difference*, London: Sage Publications.

Wrede, S. (2010) 'Nursing: globalization of a female-gendered profession' in E. Kuhlmann and E. Annandale (eds) *The Palgrave Handbook of Gender and Healthcare*, Basingstoke: Palgrave Macmillan, pp. 437–469.

Yeates, N. (2008) *Globalising Care Economies and Migrant Workers*, Basingstoke: Palgrave Macmillan.

Zinn, M.B. and Dill, B.T. (1996) 'Theorizing difference from multiracial feminism', *Feminist Studies*, 22(2): 321–331.

Zones, J.S. (2005) 'Beauty myths and realities and their impact on women's health' in M.B. Zinn, P. Hondagneu-Sotelo and M.A. Messner (eds) *Gender through the Prism of Difference*, New York: Oxford University Press, pp. 65–80.

# Index